ALSO BY GINA KOLATA

Flu: The Story of the Great Influenza Pandemic of 1918 and the Search for the Virus That Caused It

Clone: The Road to Dolly and the Path Ahead

Sex in America: A Definitive Survey (with Robert T. Michael, John H. Gagnon, and Edward O. Laumann)

The Baby Doctors: Probing the Limits of Fetal Medicine

ULTIMATE FITNESS

ULTIMATE FITNESS

THE QUEST FOR TRUTH

ABOUT EXERCISE AND HEALTH

GINA KOLATA

FARRAR, STRAUS AND GIROUX / NEW YORK

Farrar, Straus and Giroux
19 Union Square West, New York 10003

Grateful acknowledgment is made to the following people and institutions for per-
mission to reproduce the following images: The Todd-McLean Physical Culture Col-
lection, the University of Texas at Austin, for the images of Prof. W. N. Lake;
Macfadden's magazine cover; the finalists in Macfadden's 1904 contest; Emma
Newkirk; Carolyn Baumann; and the boxers Ruth Murphy and Vera Roehm. John
D. Fair for the images of Bob Hoffman, Pudgy Stockton, and John Grimek. Weider
Publications, Inc. (© July 2000) for the images of Joe Weider, and the first issue of
Your Physique. The Cooper Aerobics center for the image of Kenneth H. Cooper.
David Costill for the image of Dave Costill and Ken Sparks. Copyright © David
Hunsinger for the image of Josh Taylor. Befit Enterprises for the image of Jack
LaLanne (photographer: Maureen Donaldson). The Carson Entertainment Group for
the image of Jan Todd and Johnny Carson.

Library of Congress Cataloging-in-Publication Data
Kolata, Gina Bari, 1948–
    Ultimate fitness : the quest for truth about exercise and health / Gina Kolata.
      p.   cm.
    Includes index.
    ISBN 0-374-20477-2 (hc : alk. paper)
    1. Physical fitness.   I. Title.
RA781 .K585 2003
613.7—dc21

                                      2002192523

Designed by Jonathan D. Lippincott

www.fsgbooks.com

TO BILL, THERESE, AND STEFAN

CONTENTS

1. Less Is More, or Is It?   3

2. History Repeats Itself   25

3. How Much Is Enough?   51

4. Maximum Heart Rates and Fat-Burning Zones   73

5. Training Lore   101

6. The Athlete's World   133

7. Mount Everest   155

8. Is There a Runner's High?   175

9. Sculpting the Body Beautiful   203

10. The Fitness Business   239

    Epilogue: The Truth About Exercise   261

    Notes   269

    Acknowledgments   283

    Index   285

ULTIMATE FITNESS

one

LESS IS MORE, OR IS IT?

My friend Cynthia, just back from a week in Italy, calls me, wanting to know if I can go for a walk. She needs one, she says. She spent the day before cooped up in an airplane for endless hours and she has to have her exercise.

I am at her house in five minutes, wearing my running shorts and a T-shirt, ringing her bell, waiting while she drinks a glass of water and searches for her sneakers and puts on some sunblock. We set out, on our usual mile-and-a-half-long path. We stroll down the small hill to the end of the street, turn right, up the long hill on Edgerstoune Road. We turn left at the top, making our way into Russell Estates, an enclave of huge and showy brick houses with neatly landscaped lawns and dogs hemmed in by invisible fences. We stride around a cul-de-sac and start back, going behind Edgerstoune, on the other side of the block.

A half-hour later, we are done. Ours is a well-traveled path, one that neighbor after walking neighbor traverses daily. I see them from my kitchen window—the pairs of women, the couples, going out walking in the morning or after work. One woman even has a personal trainer who walks with her, supervising her exercise.

I live in the realm of the walking converts. Like Cynthia, they believe that walking will make them thin and fit. And if they never seem to look any different? Then, like Cynthia, they blame themselves. She tells me she has just not gotten out enough for walks. If she really kept up the program, walking daily, the exercise would do its magic, she says.

Everywhere I look, I see the walking message.

I turn on the television and the first channel that appears is showing an infomercial promoting a walking video. Smiling women give their testimonials: I was so fat I did not want them to take my picture when I went on a cruise, one says. When I heard "walking," I thought, "I can do that," she adds. Now thin and proud, she goes on another cruise, and seeks out the photographer. A former Olympic swimmer, Janet Evans, appears, wearing long black pants, slender and smiling. She, too, walks, she announces.

I pick up *Self* magazine. There it is again. Walking. Why are Americans so fat and people in other countries so slim, a story asks. It's because everyone else walks so much more. To prove it, the magazine put pedometers on a few Americans and people from a variety of places like Athens, Aibaci (in Niger), and Paris. Of course, there were some glaring economic disparities that played a role, but, sure enough, the Americans were not taking as many steps. Pauline Chu-Collins from Tustin, California, walked 4,776 steps in a day, the magazine reported. She had breakfast in bed, drove to lunch and the market, and shopped for forty-five minutes, she said. But Maria Kostaki in Athens, a bartender, put in 28,879 steps, and Ramatu Ahmad Mohammad in Aibaci, who walked for two hours to visit a friend and then walked another two hours gathering palm leaves, took 14,099 steps. Even Florence Labedays of Paris put in 13,522 steps. "I don't own a car so I do most of my shopping, errands and nights out on foot," she said, adding "I also walk to and from the train each day for work."

Walking, the article claimed, not only is "a great cardio workout" but also will "tone all your leg muscles." The source? John Reich, described as "a walking coach in Houston."

Not long after my walk with Cynthia, I am in Nantucket, a trendy island off the coast of Massachusetts where you can still find wide white beaches with no lifeguards to whistle you out of the water and sand dunes where beach grass undulates in the wind. Quaintness is the motif. Houses must be made of wooden shingles that turn a soft gray in the salty air. The town's streets are cobblestone. There are no traffic lights. There are no fast-food restaurants. No camping allowed.

But there is a gym, Nantucket Health Club, and some of us go there religiously, keeping up our workout schedule, lifting weights, using the StairMasters and elliptical trainers, and even walking on treadmills on sunny afternoons when the sky is a brilliant blue and the surf beckons, endlessly walking in place while watching television sets tuned to CNN.

I am intimately familiar with this gym since exercise is my obsession.

I believe in exercise to keep my weight down and also because I discovered that if I work out really hard and for at least forty minutes, I can sometimes reach an almost indescribable state of sheer exhilaration. I don't want to call it a runner's high—I'm not sure what that is supposed to be, though many describe it as sort of a trancelike state. That is nothing like the feeling I crave.

I often wonder what my life would have been like if I had been born to be thin, naturally thin, like my neighbor Barbara, who is tall and slim, has no intention of exercising, and never gains weight. But that is not my fate and so I have taken up exercise. Vigorous exercise. Heart-pounding, sweaty exercise. I've been doing it for years, running before they invented special running shoes or sports bras. Riding a road bike before they sold bicycling helmets. I carry my running shoes with me on every business trip, always prepared to exercise. And I seek out what I call serious gyms, places where the lifting is in earnest and the equipment well maintained.

My first gym was Spa Lady, an all-female affair with pink machines and low weights. I bought a lifetime membership. "Your lifetime or theirs?" my sister asked. One evening a month the women could invite their boyfriends or husbands to join them. When the men arrived, they would lift the stacks—putting on as much weight as the machines could hold, making sure we women saw just how tame those machines were.

I've long since moved on to a serious gym, Gold's Gym, where the color motif is black and white, and where the carpeted area for exercise machines quickly gives way to a black nonslip rubber floor. This is where free weights and the benches are kept and where men and women grunt and groan as they hoist bars loaded with heavy plates, those metal disks with a hole in the middle that you stack on the ends of metal bars. Posters on the walls for a new lifting class, called Body Pump, give the heavy-metal message to women. One shows the back of a woman lifting a barbell. "Doctors Say Women Need More Iron," it says. Another depicts a woman doing a lunge, holding a barbell on her shoulders. "Macho Is Not a Gender Thing," it says. You can see real bodybuilders at Gold's Gym, and you can hear men and women making their lifting arrangements. "See you on Saturday at eleven," one man says to his friend. "One hour. Triceps."

And I've gone through the historical sequence of exercise classes—high-impact aerobics and low-impact aerobics, advanced aerobics classes where you need the instructor's permission to attend and step classes with all their variations—before settling, for the moment, on Spinning. For a few years I went every Saturday morning to a studio that offered nothing but exercise classes and a boutique selling the then-trendy thong leotards and tights and leg warmers, a sort of *Flash Dance* look. The aerobics room had a special floor, wood covered by carpet, that was slightly raised to reduce the stress on our legs as we leapt and jumped. It had a great sound system, and the mirror-lined room fairly pulsated to the rapid beat of the tapes the instructors played. That studio is gone now, a victim, perhaps, of changing times.

I also tried, and fell in love with, each exercise machine as it was invented over the past twenty years. LifeCycles. StairMasters. Elliptical trainers. I listen to CDs of fast music when I'm on the machines—I buy them from a company that sells them to exercise instructors. I am a member of the company's frequent buyer program, getting CDs with the highest beats per minute mailed to me automatically whenever they make a new one.

But for now, my aerobic passion at the gym is Spinning. It is an industry unto itself—with its own special training programs for instructors and trademark protection so stringent that only an official forty-minute class that is conducted according to the company's specifications is entitled to be called Spinning. It also is an intense workout on a stationary bike that attracts a greater proportion of the people who are serious about exercise than most group sessions.

This morning, the Nantucket Health Club has a special event—a Spinning class, but in this case called a Spinning "event" since it is not really an official trademarked class. It costs $25, payable in advance, and the word is that it is going to be an insane workout.

I sign up and appear with my water bottle and heart-rate monitor, ready to go at nine a.m. I spot my assigned bike, number eight out of the ten stationary bikes in the room. Each bike has a small white towel draped over its handlebars.

The class is sold out, I notice. The exercisers start coming into the small Spinning room about ten minutes before the class starts, at which time the door will be closed, barring any late arrivals. We set up our bikes, arrange the seats and handlebars, put our water bottles in the special cages, strap the special watches that display our heart rates to the handlebars.

At a minute to nine, our instructor makes his entrance. Gregg D'Andrea. He looks promising. He is short, deeply tanned, and intensely muscular. His legs are shaved like those of a real bicyclist, who rid their legs of hair, they say, to make it easier to clean up scrapes when they fall. Gregg wears skintight black shorts that barely cover his crotch. He tugs on them constantly as they bunch up around his bulging glutes. His cropped, sleeveless black shirt says "Groovy" on the front and "Sex on Wheels" on the back. On his right wrist are two bracelets made of heavy links of silver. On his head, an orange bandanna.

This is the realm of the exercise aficionados. This sort of special class, with its aggressively fit instructor, is the place where you are most likely to find people who never got the message that it is okay to go slow, that you don't have to sweat to get in shape, that walking isn't just for wimps. We want to be pushed harder than we could ever push ourselves. We want to watch our heart rates climb as high as they can go, and stay there. We want Gregg to play fast techno music to set a pace, and we want him to force us to ride our stationary bicycles for forty minutes while he perches on a bike on a small platform at the front of the room, tossing his head from side to side and pedaling furiously, glistening with sweat. We don't want the usual Spinning instructor's reassurances: It's your ride. Take a break if you need one. Slow down if your heart rate gets too high.

In a way, Gregg's Spinning session is a throwback to the early days of the fitness movement. The days of no pain no gain. Of going for the burn. Now, the movement seems kinder and gentler. Walking. Yoga. Signs on aerobic machines at gyms informing exercisers of the maximum number of minutes they can stay on: "Twenty Is Plenty." Machines that measure your heart rate and warn you if the number of beats per minute goes higher than a formula allows. "Fat burning" exercises that are done at a very low level of intensity, the theory being that working harder makes you lose, if anything, *less* weight.

Gregg, explains the pale and solemn young man behind the desk at the health club, "is a breed unto himself." Every other Spinning instructor, he tells me, is tamer. The instructors have been taught not to push so hard. Gregg "is not for everyone," the young man warns.

An e-mail arrives at my computer at the *New York Times* that seems to confirm the walkers' philosophy. If what the publicist is saying is true, then maybe science is telling us that the less-is-more movement is on the right track. I may love pushing myself until my heart is pounding and my face is red with blood and my body is soaked with sweat; but that does not mean that there is any scientific evidence that this extreme notion of exercise is best. It might be that Gregg and his class—and the fact that Gregg actually told us to go for the burn—are as anachronistic as the "Groovy" on Gregg's shirt.

The press release gets right to the point: "Less is more when it comes to health and exercise, according to a new study's findings, which are going to be unveiled later this month at a prestigious exercise physiology conference in Finland," the publicist wrote.

"The effectiveness of traditional exercise programs, which usually consist of long periods of aerobic activity, aimed at achieving and sustaining a narrow target heart range, followed by a single 'cool down period,' [is] being questioned by a group of researchers from Harvard University Medical School, Columbia University College of Physicians and Surgeons, and the U.S.-based Dardik Institute." I have never heard of the Dardik Institute, but the medical schools named in the press release are, of course, among the best in the world.

The study involved healthy women ages thirty-two through fifty-eight, who exercised in very short bursts by running in place on a trampoline or pedaling on a stationary bicycle. Following one minute of exertion, they recovered for seven minutes.

"In one month, the women only did 40 minutes of actual exercise (all of it low impact)," the e-mailed press release says. And the results? "The women exhibited dramatic increases in their cardiovascular fitness and the strength of their immune systems while experiencing significant decreases in stress and anxiety."

The study, the publicist informs me, "calls into question the entire 'Aerobics Industry.'" Do I want more information? Of course, I tell him.

Okay. Why deny it? I'm a skeptic, conditioned by long years of science reporting. Why believe this report when its conclusions seem contrary to the position of the American College of Sports Medicine? The College says that aerobic endurance training for fewer than two days a week at less than 40 to 50 percent of maximum effort and for less than ten minutes "is generally not a sufficient stimulus for developing and maintaining fitness in healthy adults."

Of course, the College could be mistaken, but since it based its conclusions on a body of evidence, and since its statement was written by the country's leading experts, I had a feeling that the new study, not the college, was the more likely to be wrong. I'm also a skeptic because, like every other science reporter I know, and like many of the nation's most renowned scientists, I've been burned. I've written stories only to learn that the studies I'd based them on, often published in the world's best medical journals, contained fatal flaws and that their conclusions were wrong. And I've had scientists tell me of their own realization that they had fallen in love with hypotheses that were later disproved by more rigorous studies.

"This was the biggest disappointment of my career," said Charles Hennenkens, a Harvard researcher who had invested nearly two decades of his life in a theory that beta carotene could prevent cancer and heart disease, only to find that it didn't.

"We deceived ourselves and we deceived our patients," said Dr. Gabriel Hortobagyi, a cancer specialist at the M. D. Anderson Cancer Center in Houston, who spent years convinced that the way to fight advanced breast cancer was to give the highest possible doses of powerful chemotherapy drugs.

So as I scan the press release for this new less-is-more exercise study, I am looking for reasons why I should not believe it. My first thought is that something has to be wrong.

When you work at a place like the *New York Times*, you can count on getting hundreds of press releases every week, zinging at you by fax, e-mail, Federal Express, and regular mail. Then you get repeated phone calls. Did you receive the press release? The invitation to the press conference? The information for dialing into the teleconference? You get the tip sheets from medical and scientific journals that come out every month, some every week,

in which the editors summarize in the most enticing way the conclusions of the papers they are publishing. If you are to survive,
you have to learn to skim over these appeals and pick out the one
in a hundred, or fewer, that actually look promising.

I have another reason, as well, for being suspicious. From
what little I have seen of the exercise field, the tiny pearls of good
science are buried in mountains of junk—hucksters who promote
programs with not even a pretense of objective evidence that their
methods work; studies that involve a handful of people and have
no valid data but draw grandiose conclusions; exercise theories
that are akin to urban legends.

I expect that this new study will likely fall into one of two categories. Either it will be a reasonable piece of research that will
show that fitness does not require much effort. Or its data will be
inadequate to show anything at all. In either case, I am definitely
interested. I am aware that even if the study fails to show that less
is more when it comes to exercise, that would not be evidence
that more is more, that my maximum-sweat, maximum-effort
regimens are the right way to go. So why not take a look at this
new study, I decide. No matter how it turns out, it promises to be
a case in point.

The material arrives on a Saturday, sent via Federal Express to
my home. I tear open the box, pull out a video and press kit. The
sixteen-minute video, a cover letter informs me, was used to explain the study to its participants. I turn on my television set and
slip the cassette into the VCR.

The video begins by establishing the credentials of the researchers. The announcer says that the study will be conducted at
"the world-renowned Columbia Presbyterian Medical Center in
New York City and Hunterdon Medical Center in Flemington,
New Jersey." Then, he says, "let's meet our outstanding study researchers."

They are introduced in turn, dressed in business suits, shown giving scientific lectures, looking nothing if not professional. There also is something a bit intimidating about them. Who are we, the lay audience, to question such authority figures? Their credentials are impressive.

There is Dr. Ary Goldberger, who "heads the research team," the video says. He is an associate professor at Harvard University and also directs the Margret and H. A. Rey Laboratory for Non-linear Dynamics in Medicine at Beth Israel Deaconess Medical Center. Then there is Dr. Irving Dardik, dressed in a black suit with a white shirt and striped tie, a middle-aged man who gestures with his hands while his eyes look straight into the camera. Dr. Dardik, the video announcer explains, is a vascular surgeon who has "served as chairman of the U.S. Olympic Sports Medicine Council, where he was responsible for the science behind world-class athletic performance." Dr. Dardik, it turns out, was the inspiration behind the study. "The clinical trial will be testing his Heart Waves concept, which describes how the interaction of the human body with a novel exercise protocol with computerized feedback may impact health and possibly prevent or even reverse certain chronic diseases."

The others on the team have equally stellar credentials: Dr. Herbert Benson, also a Harvard professor, who runs the Mind/Body Medical Institute at Harvard Medical School ("Over four million of his books on mind-body medicine are printed," the announcer claims); Dr. George Stefano, who is a distinguished teaching professor at the State University of New York in Old Westbury and has written more than 240 papers published in peer reviewed journals; and, finally, Dr. Rochelle Goldsmith of the Division of Circulatory Physiology at Columbia University's College of Physicians and Surgeons.

The study will involve healthy people and also people with chronic fatigue syndrome and those with congestive heart failure, a serious, usually fatal disease in which the heart is increasingly unable to pump hard enough to supply the body with blood.

Dardik explains the theory behind the research: "In nature

you see the rhythms of nature throughout," he says. "Heart Waves recognize that the heartbeat actually climbs up and down by behavioral cycles, anxiety and relaxation, exercise and recovery. It speeds up and slows down, like coming up and down a mountain on a bicycle. Up and down. Like a roller coaster of your heart." It is, he says, "the way it works in nature. You see the rhythms of nature throughout. Everything is spiraling and cycling in the universe."

Goldberger appears on the screen: "The Heart Waves clinical trial is an exciting new adventure and it is an attempt to try out an exciting hypothesis about exercise," he enthuses.

But what do people actually do in this exercise study? The video soon shows us. A plump woman wearing gray surgical scrubs gets on a mini-trampoline. Dr. Dardik instructs her to jog slowly for about a minute, then to sit down and relax for about five minutes while her heart rate returns to normal. That, repeated several times, is the experimental program.

Dardik then explains his Heart Waves concept again.

"It's the way we actually behave, and the way we should behave and work within the context of nature's rhythm. It's natural. It makes common sense. And it's simple. But the most important thing is when you put those three together and realize how it works. It's useful. It's practical."

As he speaks, the video shows drops of water striking a blue pool, one by one, with ripples spreading outward.

But what will this exercise program accomplish? Dardik tells us.

"As you get older, your max heart rate drops. Well, suppose we have a way over time to reverse that," he postulates. "Physiologically, you'll get younger; and, also physiologically, a younger physiology can prevent disease as well. That's healthy." He describes how the wavelength of the heart's rhythm is increased. "Instead of this," he says, moving his hands up to describe a gentle slope, "you go *there*." His hands move again, describing a steeper slope.

It makes no sense to me. If you ask me what Heart Waves is, I still could not tell you. I have no idea what Dardik is saying. All I know after watching that video is that the study participants are going to exercise very briefly and then rest for a long time.

So I turn to the paper. It is an unpublished manuscript, written in the traditional format for a medical journal. "Implementation of a Novel Cyclic Exercise Protocol: Short-Term Impact on Healthy Adult Women," it is called. It includes an abstract, it lists key words for indexing, it has an introduction, a methods section, and a section called "Study Design" that describes in detail how the research was conducted. A section called "Results" follows that. Then comes a discussion section, the acknowledgments, the references, and tables and graphs of the data.

The discussion section indicates that the results were promising: "We find that a short (eight-week) course of this protocol in healthy adult women was associated with evidence of improved cardiorespiratory fitness and autonomic function, as well as subjective assessment of quality of life."

The problem is that while it has all the trappings of a scientific paper, I strongly suspect that there is almost no science there. I ask a statistician for an expert opinion. David Freedman is a professor at the University of California at Berkeley and he has written papers and books on the design and evaluation of clinical studies. He agrees to take a look at the manuscript.

I fax it to him. Two days later, he calls me, decidedly unimpressed by the study. "It is quite unconvincing," he says.

Almost everything that can be wrong with a study seems to be wrong with this one. First of all, there were only eleven women, ten of whom completed the study. From the data on these ten, the investigators managed to build a complicated, and almost impenetrable, statistical analysis, one that is "almost impossible to reconstruct from this paper," Freedman says. And from that analysis they reach their conclusion that their program was making a difference.

In preparing their analysis, the investigators apparently looked at quite a few outcomes but chose only those that seemed to point in the right direction. And there was no control group—no group of observed subjects who did not participate in the program. Without such a group, there is no way of knowing whether the changes the researchers claim they found would have occurred anyway.

Even if you take their conclusion at face value, Freedman tells me, all they have found is that the women's maximum oxygen consumption increased slightly. Was that due to the exercise? The relaxation? The alternating exercise and relaxation? The time of day? "It's impossible to say," Freedman asserts.

To be fair, I decide to show the paper to a second statistician. And I know just the person: Howard Wainer, who worked at that time at the Educational Testing Service. Not only is he well versed in the design and analysis of clinical trials, but he has a particular interest in exercise. He swims every day at lunchtime and has swum marathon distances, including the English Channel. Send the paper on, Wainer tells me.

It does not take him long to reach his conclusions. The paper, Wainer says, is impossible to interpret. There is no control group that did not have the exercise program, there is no random assignment of subjects to have the exercise program or not, and so, he says, there is no way to decide whether there was an effect, and if so, how large it was.

The investigators, Wainer adds in an e-mail to me, compared the women's fitness at the beginning of the study to their fitness at the end to argue that they saw an effect. "This is only sometimes okay," he says. "Consider using this methodology to study the efficacy of eating Cheerios for breakfast as a treatment for shortness, and using a bunch of six-year-olds as a control group: 'The study lasted a year and we found an average height gain of four inches.' " Such an analysis, he says "is okay if the (unobserved) assumption of 'no change otherwise' is true. This assumption is what the control group is for."

Finally, Wainer tells me, the investigators did twenty-three statistical tests looking for something that would turn up positive to serve as an indication that the treatment had an effect. The likelihood that, by chance alone, one of those tests would be positive is 66 percent. But that does not mean that it is a real effect; positive results showing up in this fashion are likely to be a statistical fluke. The investigators should apply statistical methods to correct this problem, Wainer maintains. But if they had made such a correction, he calculates, they would have ended up with no effect at all.

By now, I am becoming fascinated with this paper. I have to unpeel this onion. Why did anyone do this study? Why are they announcing it with such fanfare and hiring a publicist to offer it to me on an exclusive basis—a well-honed publicist's trick to try to get a journalist's attention. Is there a marketing connection in here somewhere?

The first clue comes when I notice that the paper's second author, Irving Dardik, M.D., is listed as being with LifeWaves International of New Jersey. The next clue is the video. It is produced by VHA, described in the publicist's cover letter as "the nationwide network of community-owned health care organizations and their affiliated physicians." VHA also is mentioned in the paper, as helping to pay for the Heart Waves research.

I check the VHA Web site and learn that it is a for-profit organization whose doctors and medical centers sell various products. It is a publicly traded company, I learn by checking the Securities and Exchange Commission's Web site.

Is VHA selling the Heart Waves program? Is it actually promoting this cyclic exercise as a commercial product, based on only one preliminary study of eleven women—one of whom dropped out? A study that two leading statisticians say is ludicrous?

I e-mail the publicist. I tell him that although, as he knows, I have decided not to write about the Heart Waves study for the

New York Times, I am looking into it for a book I am writing. And so, I say, I have a few questions about the groups that are participating in it: What is the relationship between VHA and LifeWaves International? Is VHA selling Dardik's Heart Waves treatment?

He replies the next day. VHA, he tells me, has invested in Life-Waves and has contributed more than half a million dollars to the research on cyclic exercise. In addition, he says, LifeWaves is about to open LifeWaves centers in three VHA hospitals in New Jersey, where people can get the Dardik program, for a fee.

But this is just the beginning of LifeWaves' plans, the publicist tells me. It expects to be opening more LifeWaves centers in VHA hospitals around the country. And, he writes, "the company will be offering individuals the opportunity of doing it themselves via a 'smart' heart rate recorder (called the LifeWaves Personal Coach) and the Internet." He makes me a special offer, to be part of the beta test of the LifeWaves Personal Coach. "It was my recommendation that they invite a very select number of media to try it and experience the results for themselves," the publicist writes.

My suspicions more than confirmed, I probe further. Page four of the study says, "This protocol was adapted from the Life-Waves Program (LifeWaves International, Califon, N.J.; U.S. Patents 5752521 and 5810737)."

Now that is interesting.

I speak to David Saloff, the president of LifeWaves International, who tells me that the company began in 1999, when Dardik's wife, Alison Godfrey Dardik, called him and asked for his help in setting it up. Saloff had known the Dardiks for about six years and had been impressed with the Heart Waves concept. Saloff tells me that he expects that most of LifeWaves' business will be with individuals and families who buy the special heart-rate monitor and the program instructions and a personalized Web page that will store the data from their workouts. People who prefer not to use the Internet can pay to get the same training at a hospital's wellness center.

But, I ask him, doesn't he want to wait for something more conclusive than the preliminary study with ten women, a study that really does not show much, if anything, about the program's beneficial effects? No, he replies. "We're talking about exercise here. I feel perfectly comfortable with it," Saloff says. All sorts of people have used the program, including elderly people with Parkinson's disease, he tells me. "There's never been an adverse event. And this, in fact, may be a safer way to exercise."

My next impulse is to check the Patent Office's Web site to see what the LifeWaves patents say. What is this new invention, and what does Dardik, in his patent application, think it does?

The first, number 5752521, is for a "therapeutic exercise program," and it was issued on May 19, 1998, at about the same time that LifeWaves International was formed. It describes the program being tested in the study but has some sections that seem, to put it mildly, a bit odd. To take just one of many examples, the patent states that "The theory underlying my invention is that the interactions which take place in the human organism and involve the biochemistry of the organism and the behavior of its organs is based upon wave communication, and not on the complexity of the organism itself." Then it gives "examples of wave activity." They include this one:

"The hunting of animals in the wild is cyclic in nature, reflecting the spike to which I have referred. Animals in the wild rarely have chronic diseases. However, when placed in zoos or domesticated, the wave patterns are flattened and become less responsive, and the incidences of chronic diseases then rival those of humans. It is also now generally recognized that chronic diseases and behavioral disorders, such as asthma, suicide, depression, criminal behavior, and cancer are dramatically on the rise."

The application goes on to provide "examples of treatment." It turns out that Dardik has much more in mind than simply helping people get physically fit. The examples he cites are of sick people made well, he claims, by his therapeutic exercise program:

A fifty-nine-year-old leukemia patient, whose elevated white blood cell count—a manifestation of the cancer—fell precipitously. A thirty-year-old woman with multiple sclerosis whose symptoms disappeared. A twenty-eight-year-old woman with AIDS who had been suffering from symptoms of severe immune deficiency for a year and a half. Within a few months of starting the Heart Waves program, "all symptoms disappeared," the patent says. An eighteen-year-old with brain cancer who, after surgery to remove the tumor, was, the patent application states, "disoriented, sleeping 18 hours a day, short term memory deficit, etc." He followed the Heart Waves program for three years, the patent application says, and "there has been no evidence of tumor recurrence."

The second patent, number 5810737, issued on September 22, 1998, is more of the same, a continuation, in fact, of the previous patent. It has many of the same sections, including the one about the animals in nature and the non sequitur about increased rates of chronic diseases and behavioral disorders. It even has the exact same descriptions of the patients who were treated with the program. This time, however, the Heart Waves program is to be synchronized with "an internal wave produced by a biological clock."

Who, I wondered, is this Irving Dardik, inventor of this unusual program?

He says he is the founding chairman of the United States Olympic Sports Medicine Council. He says he is a vascular surgeon. I search for the United States Olympic Sports Medicine Council but can find no mention of it on the Internet or in Nexis, an electronic database of published newspaper and magazine articles. Except, of course, a few stories that mention Dardik and state that he founded it.

I look on the Web site of the United States Olympic Committee. It's not there, either. So I send the Olympic Committee an e-mail asking if they ever heard of the Sports Medicine Council. A few days later they reply.

It turns out that the Sports Medicine Council really did exist, but it is now called the Sports Medicine Advisory Committee and it advises the Olympic Committee on sports medicine. Dardik was a doctor for the Olympics and was active with the U.S. Olympic Committee for about a decade, starting around 1974. So maybe my skepticism is unfounded.

But then I discover that Dardik has a very interesting history.

The story emerged in documents from a hearing before the State of New York Department of Health State Board for Professional Medical Conduct. Five patients who had multiple sclerosis testified that Dardik had told them that his "wavenergy" program would cure them. They were impressed by his credentials as founding chairman of the United States Olympic Sports Medicine Council and by an article published in *New York* magazine that lavishly praised his wave theory. When they went to Dardik, he treated them with cycles of exercise and rest, just like the subjects in his fitness study. And he charged them prices ranging from $30,000 to $100,000.

On March 22, 1995, the New York board issued its conclusions about the Dardik case. The board's Hearing Committee actually questioned Dardik's sanity, writing: "The path taken by Respondent in trying to gain acceptance for his theory as well as his deviations from proper patient care led this Hearing Committee to wonder about Respondent's mental health. Yet despite extensive use of made-up words, such as wavenergy, superlooping, matterspacetime, and frequent loose associations and expansive digressions in response to questions, the Respondent could always return to the subject when prompted and he retained the capacity to understand the questioner (usually a member of the panel) in an objective manner."

The committee added, however, that its task is to decide whether, as a doctor, Dardik "followed standards of patient care he was well familiar with from his practice of vascular surgery." He did not, the group concluded, and it revoked his medical license in New York. The board found him guilty of fraud, exercising undue influence, guaranteeing satisfaction or a cure, and failing to maintain adequate records. Dardik appealed, citing among other things the committee's allusions to his mental state as evidence it was biased against him.

The Appeals Board saw otherwise. "The Hearing Committee has the authority to assess all witnesses for their credibility. A review of a witness's behavior on the stand would properly be included in such an assessment," it wrote, adding that the committee also has the authority to direct a respondent to submit to an examination to determine mental impairment. "In this case, the Committee mentioned they had a question over the Respondent's mental state, but after review found no reason for concern."

In the end, the Appeals Board agreed with everything the hearing committee had decided. Dardik would have to surrender his medical license, it determined. The Appeals Board also imposed a forty-thousand-dollar fine, "because we feel such a penalty is the appropriate penalty for a physician who exploits several patients." It added that Dardik's conduct demonstrates "a pattern of improper and intentional mistreatment of his Patients that deserves the most severe sanctions possible."

And even though Dardik's LifeWaves International has its headquarters in New Jersey, when I check the New Jersey Medical Examiner's Web site for his name, I find his medical license has also been revoked in New Jersey.

I have to admit that I am stunned. I thought that the study that was being pitched to me was likely to be inadequate. I thought it was probably being promoted to market a product. But I never expected to uncover such an intriguing story. I had this idea that I would just deconstruct a marginal piece of research and show how hard it can be for the uninitiated to distinguish between good science and bad. I thought that I would just try to make the point that having a group of scientists from stellar institutions like Harvard Medical School and Columbia University's College of Physicians and Surgeons is no guarantee that their conclusions are to be believed.

Publicists who are trying to get reporters to write about their clients usually succeed in getting something published, I've found. So I do a quick search for the less-is-more exercise study. Sure enough, I find it, a story put out by Business Wire, available on the Internet through Yahoo! Finance. "Only Sixty Minutes of Cyclic Exercise Per Month Shown to Profoundly Affect Health," it is titled. Not only does it quote Dardik going on about his theory, but it quotes Goldberger, the Harvard researcher, about the promising results.

"This study is exciting to us," he says, "because it presents the first evidence that a novel cyclic protocol designed to train both the activation and recovery phases of exercise may increase cardiovascular fitness, increase heart rate variability, and enhance mood in healthy subjects."

On the LifeWaves Web site, Lifewaves.com, I find detailed discussions of Dardik's ideas about waves and cycles, but there also is a disclaimer. The company states: "The LifeWaves™ Program is based on the work of Dr. Irving Dardik* on understanding how rhythms or waves work in the natural world." The asterisk refers to a footnote that states: "LifeWaves International, LLC, does not endorse any claims by Dr. Dardik or others on any therapeutic benefits from this or any other exercise program. Dr. Dardik has no ownership interest in LifeWaves International, LLC. He is the spouse of the CEO of LifeWaves International, LLC, Alison Godfrey." Yet, elsewhere on the Web site, the company touts its study of the ten women, claiming that LifeWaves improved their health, and it cites ongoing studies on Parkinson's disease, AIDS, and insomnia, hinting that the LifeWaves program is improving the condition of Parkinson's patients and is being tested by leading medical centers for other medical conditions, including AIDS and insomnia.

I call Goldberger. Why, I wonder, did he get involved with this research? He explains that he has long been interested in heart-rate patterns and had found that the more variable a person's heart rate, the healthier the heart. Dardik thought that Goldberger's work fit well with his own and so, Goldberger tells me, in May of 1990, Dardik paid him a visit.

Goldberger liked Dardik's notion that humans have evolved to exercise in brief spurts and was drawn to much of what Dardik was saying. "He told me about his ideas about exercise and the idea that I thought was intuitively very very appealing, that exercise has two components, activity and recovery," Goldberger says. "The traditional exercise protocols focused on the former, but in trying to make a system more flexible you want to get the system to expand and relax. What he described made a lot of sense."

A decade later, when Dardik wanted to do a study, Goldberger was still interested. He is extremely guarded in telling me what he found, explaining that it was just a study to see if the program was feasible. "It at least showed the protocol was well-accepted," says Goldberger. "And there was a positive response in terms of the physiology, and they felt better. It said that at least the protocol has some objective validity and raises the need for further study. But I would be very cautious. It's a small group of subjects."

What about the commercialization? Goldberger tells me he has nothing to do with that and has no comment. Well, does he know about Dardik's history? He does, he says, although he did not know about it in 1990. But he does not want to discuss Dardik's past.

"My role and the role of the people I work with is in testing out ideas," Goldberger tells me. "I think Dardik poses a question to the conventional wisdom. If someone has a testable hypothesis, that's where it becomes interesting."

Cynthia calls me again, just back this time from two weeks in Chautauqua, New York, where her family vacations each August. Do I want to go for a walk?

As we head out, strolling along Edgerstoune Road, I tell her the story of Heart Waves. She is taken aback.

"I can't believe it," she says, horrified by the tale I relate.

What strikes me, though, is that the only reason I uncovered this story is because I did a sort of due diligence on a press release that I probably would have rejected out of hand had that strange video not aroused my curiosity. But now, I wonder, what else is out there in the exercise arena? What can you believe, and how do you know that what you believe is true?

two

HISTORY REPEATS ITSELF

A guy I am dating calls, very excited, telling me about a new book he is reading. It's called, he says, pronouncing it laboriously, *A-air-oh-bics*. He says it is by a doctor who has figured out how much exercise you really need, and that the book includes a test to see how fit you are.

What's the test, I want to know. It turns out that you have to go as far as you can in twelve minutes. You're supposed to run, but if you can't keep it up, you can walk part of the way. To score in the excellent category, he tells me, you have to go at least a mile and three-quarters. I have to try it, immediately.

I pull on a scoop-necked black leotard and black tights, slip on my white tennis shoes, skin my hair back into a ponytail so it doesn't get in my way, put on a long charcoal-gray coat, and head off to an indoor track. It is a cold December day, with piles of grimy slush lining the streets. I had intended to spend the afternoon studying. But I am determined to show myself that my fitness is "excellent." While my outfit sounds strange today, it seemed perfectly appropriate then. It was 1970, and runners were a rare breed, and running clothes, even running shoes, were all but unheard of. Even the word "aerobics," the title of the book with the fitness test, was new, coined by the doctor who wrote it.

I arrive at the track—the only female there. A guy asks me what I am doing and I tell him about the fitness test. I am all the more motivated, now that I have an audience, to meet the "excellent" goal. I remember running around that track, watching the clock as I dashed along for twelve minutes. And, as I recall, I went a mile and three-quarters.

But what surprises me now is that I never thought to ask a single fundamental question. Who is this doctor? And how does he know that the test of excellent fitness is to run 1.75 miles in twelve minutes? Why was I so credulous? It turns out that I was not alone.

The doctor who got me onto the indoor track that blustery day was Kenneth H. Cooper. The book he wrote, the word "aerobics" that he invented, his tireless promotion of physical exertion marked the start of a new fitness movement. *Aerobics*, published in 1968, was an instant best-seller and remained on national best-seller lists for weeks. His subsequent books, *Aerobics for Women* and *The New Aerobics*, also best-sellers, did nearly as well. Sports enthusiasts and medical experts credited him with educating people about what they really needed to know to get fit. George Sheehan, a doctor and runner who inspired millions to take up the sport in the 1970s, once said, "If you read Ken Cooper's *Aerobics* you'll know more about exercise physiology than the average physician does."

David Costill, an exercise physiologist who directed Ball State University's Human Performance Laboratory for three decades and who is one of the grand old men of the field, dubbed Cooper "a preacher," not a scientist. But because he was so good at inspiring people, his message caught on. *Aerobics*, Costill says, "was just the right book at the right time."

It was a worldwide phenomenon. To this day, jogging in Brazil is called "Coopering" or "doing the Cooper." A national fitness test in Hungary is called the "Cooperteszt."

Cooper is still around, still running, still adhering to the formula for physical fitness that he advanced in the late 1960s and early seventies. So I ask him to tell me his story, to get a glimpse into the past and an understanding of the present. If there is a place to start in a quest to understand what is truth and what is quackery in the fitness world today, and to understand an exercise industry so robust that a company like LifeWaves thinks there is a market for its program, it is with the movement that grew up around Cooper.

In a way, Cooper is an unlikely exercise evangelist, plucked from near-obscurity by capricious turns of history and a talent for self-promotion. He was working for the Air Force in San Antonio in the 1960s, studying what happens to the body when people are confined to their beds. His actual assignment was to understand, and help astronauts overcome, the debilitating effects of weightlessness on their bodies.

But, Cooper says, "that was a passing interest for me. What I was really interested in was trying to develop a conditioning program for the masses whereby we can tell you how much exercise is necessary." He decided he would apply the principles of scientific inquiry to decide how much exercise people really need to be healthy, what type of exercise is most effective in building fitness, and how to compare one type of exercise, like walking, to another, like running. His questions were simple: Is walking one mile the same as running it? If not, how many more miles would you have to walk to get the same conditioning effect? No one really had a good answer.

Cooper, however, did not start by asking whether exercise was, in fact, beneficial or even why anyone would want to exercise. He was sure that it was. His goal was to prove what he already was certain was true—that exercise makes you feel good and makes you healthy. And he wanted to persuade every adult to take it up. Cooper himself exercised—running was, and still is, his favorite means. But he had seen patient after patient start an exercise program only to drop it within a few weeks. "They gave up mentally before they gave up physically," he says. So Cooper decided that the way to get other people to exercise was to find a simple way for them to figure out how much exercise was enough. "What I had to do was to bridge the gap between faddism and scientific legitimacy."

"I had some basic questions," Cooper tells me. "What type of exercise does the Air Force population really need? How can you compare different types of exercise? And how much exercise is necessary?"

"The thing that was very very important to me was to get undeniable data. A lot of it then was anecdotal," he says, referring to reports based simply on someone's observations of a few people who were exercising.

Cooper knew the answer he wanted. He reasoned that people would have to exercise until they were out of breath, making their hearts pump faster and their lungs expand. "It was obvious that aerobic exercise was really needed," he says, explaining that was what led him to invent his word for it. "Aerobic means living in air, living in oxygen. I added an 's' to the word and made it into 'aerobics.'"

The quantification of aerobics, he decided, should be based on how much oxygen people consumed while they were exercising. And so, he tells me, he evaluated people while they were walking, running, swimming, playing tennis, playing basketball, playing golf. "All kinds of exercise," he says. And he awarded points to each one, according to how much oxygen people had to consume. "The points were based on intensity and duration," he says. Was it really that precise, I ask? Well, he replies, "some we had to estimate."

His formula was simple. He established equivalents for various forms of exercise—running a mile in less than 8 minutes equals swimming a third of a mile (or 600 yards) in less than 15 minutes equals riding a bike for 5 miles in less than 20 minutes, for example. He gave people a way to gauge their fitness by how far they ran in 12 minutes: the scale went from "very poor" with a distance of less than a mile, to "excellent" with a distance of 1.75 miles or more. And he assigned points to exercise routines and goals for the number of points one should accumulate each week to get and stay fit. The people in "very poor" condition, for example, were supposed to start by earning ten points in the first week—they could, for example, walk a mile each day for five days, taking 13:30 minutes to cover that distance. At the end of sixteen weeks, they should be earning thirty points. He proclaimed, without any really sound scientific data, that anyone who earned thirty points a week would be physically fit and remain so.

Today, when we are all exhorted to walk at least twenty minutes a day, five times a week (and, we are told, it does not even matter if it is twenty minutes all at once or twenty minutes added up from snatches of walking over the day), Cooper's regimen does not sound particularly extreme. But that was at a time when the few gyms that existed catered mainly to bodybuilders, and when there were no designer exercise classes or specialized cardio machines on the order of LifeCycles or StairMasters. Special exercise clothing had not come on the market. People were running in tennis shoes. And if it can be said that exercise enthusiasms had come in waves over the millennia, the world in 1966 was in an exercise trough.

Running was such an aberration, in fact, that stories abound about the odd looks and strange reactions that people got when they tried it. Jack Berryman, a historian of exercise at the University of Washington and an avid athlete who lifts weights every day and runs on a treadmill, tells about a track coach from Pennsylvania State University who attended a physical education conference held in Dallas in the 1960s. The coach, Berryman relates, got up at six a.m. to run. He headed off in the deserted streets but hardly went half a block when some police officers pulled him over. "They thought he had robbed someone," Berryman says. "They had never seen anyone running so early in the morning. The coach explained, 'I'm jogging.' The cops said, 'Huh?' "

Cooper's ideas seemed new at the time, but when I look into them further I find that many were first stated centuries ago. And while they were accepted as gospel by the public and many doctors, scientists tell me that they were hardly very solid, nor could they be, considering the way Cooper gathered his data.

"It's amazing that we, at the turn of the twenty-first century, are faced with the same issues as at the turn of the twentieth," Berryman says. "You just want to scream. Why don't we ever pay attention? Why don't we ever listen?" Berryman finds it endlessly intriguing that history keeps repeating itself when it comes to exercise—and even more fascinating how little known this fact is.

He tells me that the best way to understand Cooper, the exercise movement he helped start, and the exercise industry it has become today, is to go back in history and look at some ideas that started with the ancient Greeks. It is a history of exercise fads and enthusiasms, often accompanied by gnawing fears that exercise could be dangerous, even deadly.

It should be no surprise that the ancient Greeks, who worshiped the human body, were the first to write about fitness training. But for the Greeks, and for the Romans who adopted their concepts, bodily perfection was not just an aesthetic. Starting with Herodicus, a fifth-century-B.C. Greek wrestling and boxing instructor who wrote of "therapeutic gymnastics," describing exercise as a form of medicine, the Greeks and Romans believed that exercise was everyone's obligation to preserve health. Those who were athletes could take their physical development even further, with the help of trainers and coaches who devised special exercises and regimens. Much of their advice has a familiar ring.

Does regular exercise prevent disease? Herodicus certainly thought so, according to historians like Berryman, who adds that Herodicus was free with his advice on how to exercise, how much, and what benefits it would bring. Doctors, Herodicus instructed, had a duty to practice preventive medicine, not just attempt to cure the sick. His own specialty was something he called "gymnastic medicine," exercises for people of different ages and fitness levels that also took into account such things as the climate and the season of the year. He found a receptive audience in the general public, although he was opposed by physicians of his time who accused him of poaching on their territory.

"There was a big debate between the gymnasts and the physicians over whose bailiwick exercise was," Berryman says. Gymnasts, he adds, were the equivalent of today's physical education teachers or personal trainers at gyms.

But even though many physicians resented Herodicus, some heeded his words, including Hippocrates (famous for writing the Hippocratic oath). In fact, historians believe that Herodicus's most lasting effect was on Hippocrates, who wrote two books on health, published around 400 B.C. One was titled *Regimen in Health* and the other called simply *Regimen*.

In *Regimen in Health*, Hippocrates placed enormous emphasis on preventive medicine; and that, he told his readers, included exercise. He advocated walking, slowly in summer and quickly in winter, and gave advice to athletes in training.

"Eating alone will not keep a man well," Hippocrates said. "He must also take exercise." Hippocrates told people to take "sharp runs so that the body might be emptied of moisture," and to walk after dinner. "Health ensues when exercise and food are perfectly balanced." When the balance is off, people become ill.

Hippocrates, in turn, had a great impact on another influential Greek doctor, Galen. Writing in the second century A.D., Galen, who was physician to the gladiators—as well as to the Roman emperors Marcus Aurelius and his son Commodus—left a body of work that remained a leading source of Western medical wisdom for centuries, at least through the Renaissance. Galen himself had been sickly until the age of twenty-eight, when he discovered "the art of health." Exercise was a large component. In *On Hygiene*, his book for laypeople, he addressed the questions of who needs to exercise (everyone from the age of infancy on, he said) and what should count as exercise.

"To me it does not seem that all movement is exercise, but only when it is vigorous," Galen wrote. But one person's vigorous exercise might be easy for someone else, he realized, so he had to give his readers guidance in determining if they were exerting themselves hard enough. The key, he decided, is that vigorous exercise is exercise that makes you breathe hard. "If anyone is compelled by any movement to breathe more or less fast, that movement becomes exercise for him," an approach that sounds very much like what Cooper promoted in the late twentieth century.

Galen remained influential for centuries. He was studied in European medical schools in the thirteenth century as part of the revival of the teachings of the ancient Greeks and Romans. In the sixteenth century, his writings were so popular and were so often invoked by doctors that one historian called that time "the golden age of Galenism."

But it was not until halfway through the sixteenth century, in 1553, that a doctor took it upon himself to write a book entirely devoted to exercise. In his *Book of Bodily Exercise*, Christobal Mendez, a Spanish doctor, recommended exercises for both men and women—walking, he said, is best—as well as ones for young people and even the handicapped. "To preserve health, we must do our exercises," Mendez advised. His motto was "leisure hurts."

Eventually, some exercise books became best-sellers. One such text, *An Essay of Health and a Long Life*, by British physician George Cheyne, who was a member of the Royal Society, was first published in 1724; by 1745 it had gone through ten editions and was translated into French, Dutch, Latin, and German. Cheyne himself had gotten enormously fat, weighing 445 pounds, before turning to exercise. He told his readers which exercises were best. Walking, he said, was "most natural" and "most useful."

The eighteenth and early nineteenth century was an age when exercise contests became a form of mass entertainment in Europe and, later, in the United States. Men, women, and even children from all walks of life joined in, and these events would be attended by audiences numbering in the thousands.

But they were different from today's athletic events, according to Peter Radford, a professor of sports sciences at Brunel University in West London. Instead of being races in which the winner was the first to cross the finish line, these contests were carefully defined wagers. Contestants bet on how far or how fast they could run or walk—on whether or not they could run from one point to another within a specified time. There were no personal bests or record times; that was not the object.

"There was no need to run faster than the time set for the wager," Radford explained. In fact, he adds, "For the few regular racers there was the additional reason of not revealing how fast you could run, as this would affect the next wager you might make. Bets were also laid on the result of races while they were in progress, another reason for not revealing too much too soon."

Accounts of races often did not include the ages of the contestants; many just described them as "young boys" or "old men." But Radford was able to find reported ages of twenty-five men who competed in sporting events in Great Britain in that era. The youngest was a twelve-year-old boy but nearly two-thirds of the men were at least fifty years old. Some of the men's ages seem exaggerated, however, like a Richard Brown, who "was reported to be 114 when he ran 24 miles in eight hours in 1794." Or Donald McLeod, "who was variously reported to be 102 and 104 when he ran 10 miles in two hours and 23 minutes in 1790." Radford adds that McLeod "had walked from London to Inverness and back again the previous year, a distance of 1,148 miles, and astonished everyone with his 'hilarity of disposition' and 'healthful appearance' in doing so."

Fat men competed, too, even in running contests. A Mr. Hardwicke ran twenty-five miles, from Worcester to Birmingham, in 1790 in six and three-quarter hours. Newspapers reported that the event was remarkable "because of his 'gross habits of body

and unwieldy size,' " Radford says. In some events, thin men
wore weights to handicap themselves when they raced against fat
men. Young men weighted themselves down to compete equally
against old men. One thin man wore a 58-pound pad for a five-
and-a-half-mile race in 1790 and, in 1796, a twenty-five-year-old
man wore a 35-pound weight in a 10-mile race against a sixty-
year-old.

Women, young and old, also competed, often before huge
crowds. A thirty-six-year-old accepted a wager to run 30 miles a
day for 20 days, a seventeen-year-old attempted to run 40 miles a
day for 6 days. And, Radford reports, "In 1823, a girl of about
11 years managed to run alongside a professional runner in an
11-mile event, despite having to run home with her clogs after
two miles and being impeded by a crowd of boys, one of whom
she had to fight."

One of the youngest competitors was Emma Freedman of Suf-
folk, England, known as "the Pedestrian Girl." She was eight in
1823, when she competed in four contests in nine weeks: she
went 30 miles in each of the first three and, in the fourth, she was
said to have gone 40 miles in seven hours fifty minutes.

Old women also were reported to have been champion athletes. Radford tells of a seventy-year-old woman who "attempted
to run 96 miles in 24 hours in Paisley, Scotland. After 45 miles
when she was five miles ahead of schedule, she was arrested because the large and unruly crowd had threatened public law and
order."

A woman named Mary Wilkinson, said to be ninety years old
in 1764, walked 259 miles from County Durham to London in
five days and three hours. Another woman, Lady Butterfield,
"said she was 74 years old when she challenged 'any woman in
England seven years younger, but not a day older' because she
would not 'undervalue herself,' " Radford reports.

In addition to walking and running contests, there were bicycling races, boxing matches, rowing contests, wrestling bouts.

The richest athletic prize, an amount that went unmatched for more than 150 years, was won in 1809 by Captain Alardice Barclay, who walked 1,000 miles in 1,000 hours, pacing back and forth along Newmarket Heath on a one-mile measured course while a crowd of thousands watched. His prize of £16,000 was 320 times the national average income.

Many athletes, even champions like Captain Barclay, did not specialize in one event; he himself competed in contests ranging from a 440-yard dash to walks that went on for days.

The best of the athletes had coaches who controlled their diets and their sweats and purges. They issued directions on breathing and gave the athletes precise training schedules. They advised against drinking much water, saying that beer was best, even for women and children. For events lasting for hours or days, athletes often drank brandy mixed with water. Vegetables were frowned upon because they were too watery, and cheese and butter were forbidden because, Radford explains, it was thought that they "went rancid in the stomach." The coaches put camphorated oil in their mouths for a few minutes to bring it to body temperature, then spat it onto the athlete and rubbed it in. Training theories were shared among those who worked with runners, boxers, racehorses, and cocks.

And just as Chris Carmichael, the coach for champion bicyclist Lance Armstrong, wrote a book, published in 2000, on training to race bicycles, so a trainer, Walter Thom, wrote a book in 1813 titled *Pedestrianism, or An Account of the Performance of Celebrated Pedestrians of the Last and Current Century with a full Narrative of Captain Barclay's Public and Private Matches.* But training was somewhat different than it is now. Thom advised starting the day at five a.m. with a half-mile sprint, then walking for six miles. Breakfast, at seven, would be rare steak or mutton chops, stale bread, and old beer. Then it was time for the mid-morning walk, six miles again at a moderate pace. This was followed by a half-hour rest, and then another four-mile walk. At four p.m., the pedestrian ate dinner—the same meal as his breakfast—and then ended the day by repeating the early-morning reg-

imen, a half-mile sprint followed by a six-mile walk. Following
that, at eight p.m., the pedestrian went to bed for the night.

The goal was to repeat this schedule day after day until, two
or three months later, a pedestrian was walking twenty to twenty-
four miles each day. A month into the training, the pedestrian was
to start a program to "lose fat," mostly by sweating. That meant
wearing flannels while running four miles as fast as he could and
drinking a concoction known as "hot sweating liquor." It was,
according to Roberta J. Park, an emeritus professor of exercise
science and sport at the University of California at Berkeley, "car-
away seed, coriander, root licorice, and sugar candy boiled together with two bottles of cider until the preparation reduced to
half its original volume."

Nor was this regimen an oddity of pedestrianism or confined
to Great Britain. Athletic training manuals published during the
entire nineteenth century in Europe and America advocated similar programs.

America's leading walker emerged a half century later. In
1867, Edward P. Weston—"Weston the Pedestrian"—won
$10,000 in a wager that had him walking from Portland, Maine,
to Chicago.

By the middle of the nineteenth century, American doctors were
sounding a surprisingly modern cry of despair. With changing
lifestyles, and more and more people moving to cities and forsak-
ing the old agrarian way of life, the population was becoming
sedentary. They simply had to get more exercise, doctors said.
Along with the admonitions to the public to exercise, there were
entrepreneurs promoting their own dubious programs. In fact,
say Berryman and Park, "Much as unqualified 'experts' still purvey their 'systems' and 'theories' today, nineteenth-century charla-
tans were ever ready to foist their views on the American public."

Exercise was promoted as being good for the spirit and character, and as almost a moral obligation. The catchword by the

second half of the century was "muscular Christianity." Historian James C. Whorton writes: "Late Victorian physicians fairly tumbled over themselves searching for character-enhancing elements within the various outdoor games and recommendations. Thus the bicycling craze of the late 1890's was greeted with ecstatic pronouncements of not only the limitless physical improvement it promised the masses but also the opportunities for spiritual and social growth it offered."

Many used special exercise equipment—swinging Indian clubs, which were weighted clubs that looked like elongated bowling pins, or working out with a "parlor gymnasium," an early version of a chest expander. This device consisted of a rubber tube with handles at each end; one was instructed to hold the handles and pull outward. Men and women were urged to employ it on any convenient occasion, exercising at their desks or while sitting at sewing machines. There was even a small-size parlor gymnasium for children.

It was a time when some women were taking up what Jan Todd, a power lifter and a historian of exercise at the University of Texas at Austin, calls "purposive exercise." She defines it as exercise that is meant not for amusement but to elicit changes in appearance and health. "Nineteenth century women picked up dumbbells, took long walks, and joined together in calisthenics and gymnastics classes for basically the same reasons women exercise today: the implicit promise of improved appearance, the quest for better health, and the desire to feel stronger and more competent." Some women carried purposive exercise much farther, becoming professional strongwomen, performing in circuses in Europe and in the United States, where they would break chains or lift heavy weights, or where they would hold heavy weights in their teeth or perform acrobatics.

In France, a strongwoman named Olga, who called herself the "Mulatto Strongwoman," had arms that French weightlifting historian Edmund Desbonnet described as "magnificent." After seeing her perform in 1887, he wrote, "I was jealous of her biceps."

The French Impressionist artist Edgar Degas painted her doing her act.

In the United States, Josephine Wohlford, known as Minerva, was famous for her astonishing strength, lifting eighteen men and a platform at one time "for a total weight of approximately 3000 pounds," Todd said. "The weight has never been approached by any other woman."

While strongwomen were not always viewed as paragons of the female form, by the end of the nineteenth century, exercise—or, more specifically, the muscles it could produce—was marketed to women as the path to beauty. One charismatic promoter, Bernarr Macfadden, who founded the enormously successful magazine *Physical Culture*, and who later, in the 1920s, went on to create the true-confessions magazine genre, told women that muscles were the key to physical attractiveness. A special section of *Physical Culture* for women, published in June of 1899, stated that "there can be no beauty without fine muscles." His motto was: "Weakness is a crime. Don't be a criminal."

In August 1900, Macfadden put a woman holding dumbbells on his magazine's cover. In October of that year, he started publishing the first fitness magazine for women, *Women's Physical Development*. Three years later, he changed its name to *Beauty and Health: Women's Physical Development*, and sales soared.

Then, in what Todd calls "a stroke of editorial and public relations genius," Macfadden announced that his magazine was sponsoring a contest with a $1,000 prize for "the best and most perfectly formed woman." The winner would be chosen on January 2, 1904, the last day of a three-day exhibition of physical fitness at Madison Square Garden that would feature running races for men and women, fencing contests, and even fasting competitions. The panel of judges who would choose the most perfectly formed woman included sculptors and doctors as well as physical trainers.

They chose Emma Newkirk of Santa Monica, California. She was five feet, four and a quarter inches tall and weighed 136 pounds. Her bust was 35 inches, her waist 25, her hips 36, and her thighs 23½ inches. Her publicity photo shows her posed like a Greek statue in a skintight union suit, which many decried as pornographic. Her hair is piled in a loose bun atop her head. Her arms are folded and held out from her chest at a right angle. Her weight is on her right leg, her left positioned behind her as if she is about to take a step. Her body, by today's standards, looks a bit chunky and lacks the chiseled muscles that female body-builders now acquire. And her pose is nothing like the muscle-defining ones that today's bodybuilders strike.

The following year, Macfadden held another contest, but this time the women had to compete in eight athletic contests: a 50-yard run, a 220-yard run, a 440-yard run, a running high jump, a two-hands lift, a half-mile run, a mile run, and a three-mile race billed as "go as you please." The winner, Marie Spitzer of New Haven, Connecticut, placed first in six of the eight athletic contests, but was rated only fourth by the judges of her body's physical development.

But by the start of the twentieth century, a movement that be-gan in the 1860s to separate amateur from professional athletes had finally changed the nature of sports. Young and middle-class men at universities began to dominate athletics, and sports that involved wagers and prizes were scorned. Eventually, betting on the outcome of athletic contests was prohibited. Collegiate sports, like football, tennis, golf, rowing, and track and field, became cel-ebrated for developing character and team spirit.

"The old sport died, and with it its culture, personalities, and achievements," Radford sadly relates.

It was replaced by a new emphasis on exercise for the improve-ment of the individual and the race. President Theodore Roo-sevelt was the exemplar at the turn of the century. He saw "action and sport as a revitalizing agent for the neurasthenic and dyspep-tic American male," writes Harvey Green, a professor of history at Northeastern University in Boston. He notes that when Roo-sevelt went on an African safari in 1909, his adventures were avidly chronicled in newspapers and even inspired a toy set,

"Teddy's Adventures in Africa," made by the Schoenhut Toy Company of Philadelphia.

Men and women alike joined gyms, including ones opened by Louis Attila, who was popularly known as Professor Attila. (His given name was Ludwig Durlacher, but he adopted the name Attila after Attila the Hun.) A strongman and trainer, he had made his reputation in Europe in the late 1800s. His first gym was in Brussels, where he discovered and trained one of the most famous strongmen of all time, Friedrich Mueller, who went by the name Sandow. Then he opened a gym in London, where his clients included the Prince of Wales.

Attila arrived in New York City in 1893, soon opening a modest gym where men and women trained together; he later opened branches in Detroit and Chicago. Then came his pièce de résistance: a gym he created in New York's theater district that was unlike anything America had ever seen. Its every detail was planned to perfection, Todd relates. "To attract the right kind of clientele, Attila knew it was important to give his gym a suitable name. A short, simple name like World Gym would not have conveyed the elegance and sophistication Attila hoped to achieve. But 'Attila's Athletic Studio and School of Physical Culture' made his members feel as if they were getting 'physical education,' not just a workout. The use of 'studio' was also significant as it conveyed the artistic aspect of building the body; it also made the facility more appealing to women." There were Turkish carpets on the floor. Replicas of Greek statues "helped create an atmosphere of elegance, refinement, and classical beauty," Todd notes. Even the barbells were elegant, with brass spheres and nickel-plated bars. At first, Attila's clients were men, including J. Pierpont Morgan, Jr., Alfred Vanderbilt, Florenz Ziegfeld, Oscar Hammerstein, John Philip Sousa, and James J. Corbett, a heavyweight boxing champion. Attila had disparaged American women, claiming that they were lazy and too obsessed with fashion and that their lack of exercise had given rise to "deformities," such as shallow chests and thin necks. But soon he changed his mind, taking on women as clients, teaching them to lift weights and box, claiming he was showing them how to "hit like men."

"Actress Edna Wallace Hopper reported that along with her dumbbell and medicine ball routine she regularly boxed with Jack Cooper while training at Attila's gymnasium," Todd reports. An undated article from *Vanity Fair* in Attila's scrapbook, titled "How a New York Woman Develops Her Figure," showed a woman in Attila's studio hitting a punching bag, boxing with a man, and working out with weights.

His most famous female student was Carolyn Baumann, who came to Attila's Chicago studio when she was eighteen, wanting to lose weight. Ten months later, she had lost 25 pounds and was astonishingly strong. The *National Police Gazette*, a sports newspaper that was sort of the *Sports Illustrated* of its time, said she was the "most magnificent specimen of womanhood in the world." Baumann, Todd says, began working for Attila, teaching boxing to society women.

"Sport historians refer to the 1920's as the golden age of sport," notes Todd. Men and women trained with Indian clubs and weights, there were professional strongmen and strongwomen. People played tennis, competed in track-and-field events, in swimming. Fitness "was a fad." And like all fads, it faded.

The movement ended with the Depression. When most people could no longer afford to belong to a gym, the obsession with strength and fitness and physical appearance of the previous decade began to seem increasingly frivolous. "When we hit the Depression, the money people had for gym memberships went for other things. The gym culture declined," Todd says. It was not until after World War II that fitness reemerged as a national issue, but this time it was for a different reason.

It began with a call to arms. A paper by Hans Kraus and Ruth Hirschland of the Institute of Physical Medicine and Rehabilitation at the New York University Bellevue Medical Center reported that 56.6 percent of 4,264 American children tested were so unfit that they had "failed to meet even a minimum standard required for health." By contrast, the report's authors found that when 2,879 children in Switzerland, Austria, and northern Italy were given the same tests, just 8.3 percent failed. The tests included sit-ups, leg-lifts (both while lying faceup and while lying facedown), and reaching down and touching the floor without bending the knees.

Kraus and Hirschland wrote that the lack of exercise among American youth was "a serious deficiency comparable to a vitamin deficiency" and that there was an "urgent need" to rectify the situation. They received national attention, even from President Dwight D. Eisenhower, who received the report from Kraus and an associate, Bonnie Pruden, a physical trainer who directed the Institute for Physical Fitness in White Plains, New York. Eisenhower said he was shocked by its findings. He held conferences and established the President's Council on Youth Fitness, headed by Vice President Richard M. Nixon. Its members included five cabinet officers.

Pruden then wrote a popular book, *Is Your Child Physically Fit?*, with an introduction by Kraus. In it, she blamed Americans' softness on their sedentary lifestyle. Parents pushed babies in strollers, then drove their children in cars instead of insisting they walk or ride bicycles, and allowed them to watch television for hours on end. In Europe, she noted, everyone walked. They climbed stairs instead of taking escalators. They ran to keep warm if it was cold outside. American youth, she added, were so out of shape that they might well be unable to endure military training, and unable to fight to defend the nation.

There were dissenters. Peter V. Karpovich, a professor of physiology at Springfield College in Massachusetts, said that the main reason American children failed the fitness test was that they could not bend over and touch the floor without bending their knees. But, he said, if children did warm-up exercises for five minutes before attempting this test, most who had failed would pass.

Military officers assured interviewers that young men who were out of shape when they joined the armed forces quickly became strong and fit after basic training.

But the report had put fitness—and exercise—on the national agenda.

One of John F. Kennedy's first items of business when he became president in 1961 was to hold a conference on fitness. In 1963, the President's Council on Youth Fitness was expanded and renamed the President's Council on Physical Fitness, to become, in 1968, the President's Council on Physical Fitness and Sports. Its mission was to promote exercise and fitness for Americans of all ages.

It was not entirely successful.

Many American men in the 1960s played golf and, inspired by the Kennedy mystique, the occasional game of touch football. Women often exercised at home, following along with national television stars like Bonnie Pruden, Jack LaLanne, and Debbie Drake, who promised them beauty, health, and attractiveness. And they bought fitness record albums that let them continue to exercise on their own.

The back cover of one of Debbie Drake's albums, *How to Keep Your Husband Happy*, told women that excess weight and slack muscles were unattractive. "Heavy, flabby arms can make a woman look much older than she is . . . There is nothing more unattractive than fat thighs. I dislike myself when my thighs get a little heavy." But she explained what women could accomplish through exercise: "There is a great reward for getting that figure back where it ought to be. Nothing is quite so good for the ego as admiring glances from the man you love. Money won't buy it and dieting and exercising will accomplish it." Exercise also would give women grace, she said. "A large part of a woman's allure to a man is in her movements. A graceful woman is like a cat. In order to have graceful, slow movements, a woman needs her strength. Her body should be strong yet give the appearance of being delicate and tender. Exercise, if done properly, does this."

Women, in particular, were concerned about their bodies in those years. Clothing styles had changed and their bodies were uncovered. "In the 1950s," notes Todd, "you see the bikini introduced. It was common to wear shorts. Halter tops were a big deal. These are big changes. So women start saying, 'Maybe I should do push-ups or sit-ups.' "

The perfect body in those years was not heavily muscled. Nor were the exercises that men and women took up strenuous. The ideal body had no obvious musculature—a sort of Cary Grant look for men and an Audrey Hepburn look for women. The sophisticated life, as portrayed in books and movies, described so vividly by writers like John Cheever, featured cigarettes and cocktails before dinner, not a sweaty session in a gym or on a tennis court or a five-mile run.

The reason was fashion and culture. In the 1960s and seventies, the youth culture and the hippie movement set the standards for beauty and fitness. "It was just uncool to be interested in exercise," Todd remarked. The aesthetic promoted a Twiggy look for women and a George Harrison look for men. Competitive sports were frowned upon. "They were challenged by the sixties movement of peace, freedom, love. The whole notion of being competitive became uncool. To be seen as a jock meant that, in certain quarters, you were stung by being not with it. You were seen as a Neanderthal."

Of course there were athletes in America in the sixties and seventies and there were many who ignored the current fads. But strenuous exercise for the most part had gone out of style.

Robert Lipsyte, a sports columnist for the *New York Times*, recalls: "In the early 1960s, still firm from Army basic training, I began swimming in a Manhattan YMCA and running in Riverside Park along the Hudson River. This was fairly aberrant behavior at the time. Such people were called 'health nuts.' Almost no one ran. In the park, I was usually alone except for an occasional boxer, who ran in combat boots and a watch cap, and stopped to snort and throw a few punches. I felt tough just running behind him."

Kenneth H. Cooper relates his experiences in the 1960s, when he urged men to exercise. They would argue with him and tell him that they did not need to work out. This, he says, was everyone's favorite excuse: "Doc, I don't need much endurance. I work at a desk all day, I watch television at night. I don't exert myself any more than I have to, and I have no requirements for exerting myself. Who needs large reserves? Who needs endurance?"

Women, according to Cooper, were even worse than men. "One of the great disappointments of my career is the general indifference of American women toward exercise," Cooper wrote in his 1968 book *Aerobics*. "American men are indifferent to it, obviously—four out of five of them are out of shape—but at least they sit home and worry about it once in a while. Women don't." He tells of a Seattle woman who, he says, was typical. "She spent most of the lecture polishing her fingernails but sought me out afterward. 'Doctor, I don't care about the heart and the lungs and all that. I just want some sweet little exercise that will keep my tummy tucked in.' "

The federal government was not keeping statistics in those days on Americans' exercise habits; that started with a report by the Centers for Disease Control in 1985. The report stated that just 15 percent of adults engaged in vigorous physical activity for at least 20 minutes three times a week and that just 22 percent engaged in physical activity of any intensity at least five times a week for 30 minutes at a time. A quarter of the population said they engaged in no significant physical activity at all. It is hard to imagine any more dismal statistics than those, and yet 1985 was a time when the country supposedly had discovered physical fitness. In the 1970s, however, Cooper says that people not only did not exert themselves but they saw no particular need to.

And if healthy people disdained exercise, people who had heart disease, and many who were at an age when they were at risk of heart attack, often harbored a mortal fear of strenuous activity. "When I was in medical school, in the 1960s, we were taught that you shouldn't exercise people over age forty," Cooper tells me. Doctors also were taught that people with heart disease must avoid all strenuous exertion and people who had just had a heart attack were supposed to rest in bed—a prescription very different from the standard practice of today, when heart attack patients are encouraged to begin exercise programs as part of their cardiac rehabilitation.

"In 1968, I said that people could jog even past forty, fifty, sixty years of age," Cooper recalled. That message met, at first, with dismay and disbelief.

Yet Cooper and a few other running evangelists had struck a chord, or perhaps it was just that the tides of fashion were ready to shift again. With their unflagging efforts to promote exercise, they helped set the stage for health clubs, aerobics classes, personal trainers, bodysculpting, special exercise gear, and magazines and books promising health and beauty through fitness.

It began with the craze for running.

One of the running movement's inspirations was George Sheehan, a family doctor in Rumson, New Jersey, a quiet little town on the Navesink River, not far from the ocean. Sheehan discovered running in the early 1960s, and soon became one of its most avid spokesmen. "At the age of 45, I pulled the emergency cord and got off the train," he wrote.

His son Andrew wrote of those early days: "Initially, he took pains to hide the fact that he was running at all. Running in public would have been viewed as subversive in a town such as ours—perhaps in any town. In the early 1960's, there was no such thing as a middle-aged man jogging down the street. Thus he began his running in the privacy of our backyard." Eventually George Sheehan took to the streets. His children were at a loss to explain him. " 'Why does your father run around town in his underwear?' we children were asked. I recall being unable to answer—recall, too, a touch of embarrassment."

By the mid-1970s, George Sheehan had become a running

celebrity, competing in marathons, contributing articles to *Running* magazine, writing best-selling books, and jibing at Flabius Americanus—the overweight American—who needed only to put on a pair of running shoes and hit the roads to learn what it truly meant to be alive. "Do your own thing, as long as it raises your heart level to more than 120 beats a minute for half an hour—four times a week," he wrote.

Along with Sheehan, there was Jim Fixx, another apostle of running, whose best-selling book *The Complete Book of Running*, published in 1978, brought multitudes of converts to the movement. Fixx repeated his message tirelessly before rapt audiences, telling them that he was the living embodiment of the glories of running. It literally changed his life, Fixx reported. He stopped smoking, his excess pounds dropped off, and, he writes, "what I found even more interesting were the changes that had begun to take place in my mind. I was calmer and less anxious. I could concentrate more easily and for longer periods. I felt more in control of my life. I was less easily rattled by unexpected frustrations. I had a sense of quiet power, and if at any time I felt this power slipping away I could easily call it back by going out and running."

Not everyone was entranced by this self-ordained running priesthood. Frank Deford, writing in *Sports Illustrated* in 1978, carped: "I am sick of joggers and I am sick of runners. I don't care if all the people in the U.S. are running or planning to run or wishing they could run. All I ask is, don't write articles about running and don't ask me to read them. I don't ever want to read about the joy of running, the beauty, the pain, the anguish, the agony, the rapture, the enchantment, the thrill, the majesty, the love, the coming-togetherness, the where-it's-atness. I don't want to hear running compared to religion, sex, or ultimate truth."

Nonetheless, the evangelism of Fixx, Sheehan, and Cooper prodded millions of American to start to run. Of course, most Americans remained sedentary, but it was hard to ignore the avid group who became running enthusiasts. Cooper says that in the early 1960s, only about 100,000 Americans identified themselves as runners, but by the late seventies that number had grown to more than 30 million. An industry sprang up to accommodate them—soon there were running shoes, running bras, running shorts, runners' warm-up suits, treadmills, running clubs, books on running, running competitions from marathons to "fun runs," and numerous running magazines. And this was for a sport that, in essence, required no equipment.

It was the start of a new era of fitness promotion. Women took aerobics classes, their popularity boosted by Jane Fonda, who released her first workout video in 1982. She told women that exercise was going to make them vibrantly healthy, and offered herself as an example. "I have always made a point of stressing that the goal of exercising and becoming fit is not to form yourself into the contours of some 'fashionable' mode, not to look like someone else, but to make your body as vibrant as it can be . . . That is what the Workout has done for me."

That same year, Reebok produced the first shoe that was specially designed for such classes. "The 1980s gave us the proliferation of athletic footwear," said Larry Weindruch, the director of communications at the National Sporting Goods Association. "That's when Nike and Reebok really came into their own." Footwear sales rose from $1.8 billion in 1981 to $6.4 billion in 1990, the industry group reports. Corrected for inflation, that is an increase of 147 percent.

Exercise classes at health clubs proliferated, with low-impact aerobics introduced in 1985, in an attempt to prevent injuries from the leaps that were part of the traditional classes. Soon gyms were featuring computer-controlled equipment, like exercise bikes and step climbers that featured variable programs. By 1990, exercise on stair-climbing machines had become the fastest growing American fitness activity, according to IDEA, an organization of health fitness professionals. Personal trainers became a presence in gyms in the 1990s, IDEA notes, adding that in 1991, the group had 791 personal-trainer members. By 2001, there were 8,000 and in 2002, according to the organization, 5.2 million Americans paid for the services of a personal trainer.

Yet with the burgeoning fitness movement came concerns: How much exercise is enough? When does exercise become obsessive? When is it dangerous to one's health? And what can be done to get the sedentary moving?

three

HOW MUCH IS ENOUGH?

Steven N. Blair used to think that the more exercise one got, and the more vigorous it was, the better. He should know. As the director of research at the Cooper Institute in Dallas, a nonprofit research center founded by Ken Cooper, it was Blair's job to study the benefits of exercise. He also put his beliefs into practice—he ran every day and even ran marathons. All along, he counseled people who came to the Cooper Institute for health advice to keep training, to keep working harder and harder. "The message was that you needed to do vigorous exercise," Blair says.

Lately he has changed his mind. And he is not alone. The story of why and how public health experts and exercise physiologists decided how much exercise is enough was the culmination of a century-long quest that focused on one organ, the heart.

It began around the turn of the last century, when doctors started talking about a newly recognized syndrome that could, they said, kill an athlete at any moment. They called it "athlete's heart."

The syndrome made sense to many concerned doctors. Athletes tended to have large hearts and irregular heart beats. They often had heart murmurs—sloshing sounds in their heart when blood that was being pumped out of the heart slipped back in again through leaky valves. These were all symptoms of heart disease, seen in patients with gravely serious medical conditions. If they were appearing in athletes, that was not good, doctors reasoned.

"To most early twentieth-century physicians, an enlarged and irregular heart with murmurs was a diseased heart, and athletes were thus easily diagnosed as casualties of their sports," according to James C. Whorton.

Even worse, some medical authorities feared that athlete's heart might be the cause of the growing incidence of heart disease. It was a time when strenuous sports were becoming increasingly popular. It may not be just coincidence, some doctors said, that more and more people were suffering heart attacks. Soon some of the very doctors who had once urged people to exercise were issuing stern admonitions against it.

The warnings started appearing in leading medical journals, written by highly respected doctors. In 1910, an editorial in the *Boston Medical Journal*, the most prestigious of its time, declared: "Every year, the death rate from cardiac disease is increasing and unless something is done to check this it will become more of a menace than tuberculosis or acute respiratory diseases."

As it gained currency, the athlete's-heart theory was elaborated by doctors into a belief that just as an athlete's biceps or quadriceps shrink and get flabby when the athlete stops training, so the heart will atrophy and grow fatty. They warned of "fatty heart" and said that athletes were courting premature death. Once people started to exercise, they got onto a ruthless treadmill: the only way to prevent the heart from deteriorating was to keep exercising, no matter how tired of exercise they might become, no matter how old they grew.

It seemed logical. When athletes competed, their hearts raced, they were breathless, and it seemed clear that their hearts were under great strain and could give out. Whorton recounts some of the alarming stories that began circulating. In an 1882 book, *Diseases of Modern Life*, a leading British public health advocate,

Benjamin Ward Richardson, wrote of seven former athletes who died young but who might "have lived to a vigorous old age under a system less lawless in nature and less suicidal." In the United States, an article published in 1905 in the *New York Medical Journal* told of an Illinois college whose varsity tennis players, claimed the school's president, were dropping dead early from athlete's heart. "Many have died of heart disease between the ages of forty and forty-five, when they should have been at their best physically."

"Mr. C.," reported a New York physician, "lived a bit longer, to the age of fifty-two, but finally the heart he enlarged through cycling turned on him after sedentary years as a bookkeeper. The weakened organ began demanding beer, then cigars, but in the end even these stimulants proved inadequate." Poor Mr. C. developed shortness of breath and chest pain upon only the mildest exertion. His heart muscle was inflamed, his heart was enlarged, his coronary arteries were stiffened and narrowed.

Some were terrified by their doctor's warnings of the harm they had done themselves by exercising. Whorton tells of an eminent Yale economist, Irving Fisher, whose doctor told him in 1896 that he strained his heart when he rode his bicycle up hills. Fisher thought he was doomed. "I feared sudden death and I feared to hear my heart beat on my pillow," he wrote.

In 1897, when the Boston Athletic Association sponsored the first American marathon, medical experts erupted in cries of alarm. The *Journal of the American Medical Association* opined that it was "unquestionable" that the marathon runners would injure their hearts. Some doctors said that marathon runners should have taken note of the first marathoner, the soldier Pheidippides, who is said to have run forty kilometers from Marathon to Athens in 490 B.C. to announce that Greece had defeated Persia in battle. When he arrived at his destination, Pheidippides dropped dead from exhaustion.

(Paul Thompson, a physician who directs the program in preventive cardiology cardiovascular research at Hartford Hospital in Connecticut, and who is professor of medicine at the University of Connecticut, writes that the Pheidippides story is a myth: "Pheidippides was more likely named Philippides or Phidipus. His run was not from Marathon to Athens to announce victory but from Athens to Sparta to solicit military aid and then back to Athens with the bad news that the Spartans were not coming. This distance was not 40 km but closer to 500 km [300 miles]. Most distressing of all to those who would cite this event, our runner, name uncertain, probably survived. Herodotus, the major historian of the event, never mentioned the runner's demise.")

A terrifying story of athlete's heart was the untimely death of William Blaikie, a member of the Harvard crew team in the mid-1860s who had subsequently become a weight lifter. In his professional life, he worked as a lawyer, but he also found time to write a best-selling book, *How to Get Strong and How to Stay So*, which was published in 1879. After he turned sixty, however, Blaikie stopped exercising. He died at age sixty-one, of a stroke, attributed to the fact that his heart degenerated when his exercising stopped.

Other sports also began to seem recklessly dangerous. Bicyclists were racing 500 miles in twenty-four hours and they were staging six-day races. In 1903, the most famous, and likely the most arduous, bicycle race, the Tour de France, began as a way for a newspaper, *L'Auto*, to sell more copies. The paper announced the race on January 19, 1903, as "the greatest cycling trial in the entire world. A race more than a month long: Paris to Lyon to Marseille to Toulouse to Nantes to Paris." Sixty riders eventually signed on for the 2,388-kilometer race (about 1,400 miles). Within a few years, the race had become even more grueling, with a course through the Pyrenees Mountains in 1910, and through the Alps in 1911.

Medical experts fretted that never before in history had athletes subjected themselves to such physical stress. Benjamin Ward Richardson wrote in a paper published in 1895 in *Medical Society Transactions* that bicyclists who competed in the twenty-four-hour races were forcing their hearts to push 200 tons of blood. He insisted that it was impossible to argue that their hearts would not be damaged by such stress. That, he wrote, "is not . . . within the realm of possibility."

Of course, there were skeptics who pointed to published surveys of former athletes that indicated that, on average, they actually lived longer than non-athletes. But fears remained, shadowing the exercise movement. Some doctors tried to gather data to refute the claims that athletes damaged their hearts. They surveyed former athletes and reported that they were fine, suffering no excessive deaths from heart failure. In 1903, George Meylan, the medical director of Columbia University's physical education program, reported in a paper published in 1904 in *American Physical Education Review*, on a study of men who had rowed for Harvard between 1852 and 1892. He compared their death rate to the average rates in life-insurance tables and concluded that they lived, on average, five years *longer* than typical American men. And, he observed, they were generally healthier, more energetic, and more fertile than other men.

Harold Williams and Horace Arnold, two doctors at Tufts Medical School, examined nearly all of the fourteen runners (all men) who completed the 1899 Boston Marathon and found that they had enlarged hearts and that they manifested heart murmurs after the race. And yet, the two doctors wrote in their report, published later the same year in the *Philadelphia Medical Journal*, these were not evidence of medical pathology. The only casuality of the race was a medical-corps member whose bicycle hit a dog while he was riding alongside the runners. Another study of Boston Marathon runners, published in 1903 in the *Boston Medical and Surgical Journal*, concluded that the most serious injury associated with the sport was blistered feet.

But fear of athlete's heart persisted, and even athletes who tried to brush off warnings about the dangers to their hearts lived in fear that the doctors might be right. That, in fact, was the fate of Clarence DeMar.

DeMar, a natural runner, describes himself in his 1937 book *Marathon* as an oddity. He dashed through New England towns and began training for his first marathon in 1909 by running the seven miles between his home and his job at a Boston area printer. Some days he would run one way only; others, he would run the round trip.

"Frequently, the men in the shops showed an interest in my way of travel," DeMar writes. "Now and then, one would advise me of the danger to heart and health. Once a man in the street offered me a dime for carfare; and again while passing through West Everett, someone yelled insistently 'Hey! Hey! you running?' I stopped. Then he said, 'A year from now you'll be dead, running like that!' "

The next year, DeMar fell in with some trainers who became his advisors. "They talked about eating plenty of meat, getting a long stride, taking breathing exercises, and having the 'guts' to fight to the finish," DeMar writes. They also took him to a doctor in Roxbury, Massachusetts, for a physical examination.

"He [the doctor] told me that I had a slight heart murmur and should not run more than a year or two. I asked him how I'd first notice anything wrong with my heart, and he said that in a few years I'd feel weak, going up and down stairs." DeMar adds that he looked for those symptoms over the next quarter of a century but they never emerged. Still, that was not the last time he would be warned.

In 1911, he entered the Boston Marathon. "Before the race, as usual, the staff of doctors examined all the contestants and advised one or two not to start," DeMar tells us. "They listened quite a while at my chest and gave the verdict that this should be my last race and I should drop out if I got tired. They said I had heart murmurs." DeMar reports that he took this advice with a grain of salt. "I do not know whether it is possible to run a marathon without getting tired," he says, "but at any rate, I've never done it." He won the race.

In 1912, DeMar stopped running marathons, in large part because all those warnings about his heart had started to weigh on him. He only took up marathon racing again in 1917, when it was increasingly likely that the United States would enter the world war, reasoning that "if I went to war I might get killed. Why not have a little fun marathoning first?"

The relentless publicity over the dangers of exercise had its intended effect, as more and more people decided that there was no point in stressing their bodies. Cardiologists said middle-aged and older people should take it easy, and heart-attack patients were advised to be wary of any exercise that would make their hearts beat fast. The concerns persisted. Middle-aged doctors today recall being taught in medical school that heart-attack patients should rest for weeks and then take it easy for the rest of their lives—a message that is very different from the consensus today. Now doctors encourage most heart-attack patients to start walking while they are in the hospital and urge them to continue exercising after they return home, to join programs that involve walking and, later, for those who can, even jogging.

It was not until the start of the exercise boom in the 1970s, that twentieth-century fears about exercise's effects on the heart began to be replaced by the fervent belief that exercise, the more vigorous the better, would help the heart and prolong life. It was a message with a turbulent start as evidenced by Cooper's reception in the late sixties, when he began advocating that almost everyone take up a regimen of vigorous exercise. And it was a message that met with resistance, countered by exercise evangelism, countered by an I-told-you-so retort by the skeptics when one famous case seemed to prove them right.

Cooper says he knew he was going to infuriate other doctors with his exercise message. To be safe, before encouraging middle-aged and elderly people to start strenuous activity, he tested their hearts, offering them stress tests. He would hook them up to equipment that monitors their heart rate, breathing, blood pressure, and their heart's electrical impulses. Then they would walk on a treadmill, slowly at first and then faster as the treadmill's speed and its incline were gradually increased until the person could not exercise any harder. The test can show how the heart handles the demands of exercise and can reveal whether obstructed coronary arteries impede the heart. In Dallas, where Cooper wanted to set up an entire center to provide stress tests and fitness evaluations, he almost was shut down before he began.

"The medical board of censors in Dallas thought I would kill people with my stress test," Cooper admitted. He won them over, convincing the group, an organization associated with the Dallas Medical Society, that the tests were safe. In fact, "the second person who came for stress testing was the chairman of the board of censors."

"In 1972, we started exercising cardiac patients," encouraging them to start mild exercise programs as part of cardiac rehabilitation. Other doctors were appalled. "They were sure I had flipped my lid by then," Cooper recalls.

Cooper advised Americans not to worry about injuring their hearts. "The athlete's heart, if different from normal, is definitely above normal." Athletes' hearts got larger because they had to supply more blood to the body. "You might think of an athlete's heart as a muscular, healthy heart," he wrote.

Many doctors were not convinced, but exercise enthusiasts soon found what sounded like a compelling argument that running was safe, and even life prolonging. They began citing the theories of Thomas J. Bassler, a pathologist who worked at the Centinella Valley Community Hospital in California and who was one of the founders of the American Medical Joggers Association. He claimed that running protected the heart to such an extent that anyone who ran a marathon in less than four hours would never have a heart attack.

His evidence was not exactly scientific. He maintained that his autopsies showed that two-thirds of Americans were dying prematurely from what he called a combination of "loafer's heart, smoker's lung, and drinker's liver." Training for a marathon forced runners to adopt a lifestyle that would protect their hearts. Most eat low-fat diets and do not smoke.

While many medical experts disputed Bassler's contentions, runners everywhere decided they must be true. Hal Higdon, a runner who writes training guides for marathons, described how Bassler repeatedly dodged his critics: "The criticism centered on Dr. Bassler's lack of evidence. He had not done a controlled study. All he had done was propose a theory and ask medical experts to prove him wrong—which was not the way serious medical research was conducted.

"Over a period of years, eminent cardiologists attempted to dispute Dr. Bassler's theory. They would cite evidence of a runner dead of a heart attack, and Dr. Bassler would point out that the runner didn't run marathons. They would cite a marathoner who had collapsed in the last mile, and Dr. Bassler would note that the runner didn't finish the race. Dr. Bassler refused to accept anecdotal evidence of coronary deaths, demanding to see X rays. In several apparent marathon coronary deaths, he identified the culprit as dehydration or a cardiac arrhythmia rather than the standard heart attack caused by blocked arteries. On several occasions, when seemingly pinned into a corner with his theory disproved, Dr. Bassler would modify the theory just enough to maintain the controversy."

In the end, Higdon writes, Bassler prevailed, at least in the minds of the general public, who became convinced that "running distances of 26 miles and 385 yards was not fraught with danger, that marathoners were not routinely collapsing, clutching their hearts, that marathon running should not be banned from city streets as a matter of public safety. Each critic of Dr. Bassler, by digging deep to uncover examples of supposed marathon deaths, inadvertently was proving what I consider to be his main message: that marathon running was a relatively safe sport and a benign activity as long as you trained intelligently, behaved rationally and took proper precautions (such as drinking plenty of liquids on hot and humid days)."

But the public's view changed quickly when they heard the shocking news of July 20, 1984: Jim Fixx, one of the leaders of the running movement, died of a massive heart attack, his lifeless body found by a motorcyclist on the side of a road in Hardwick, Vermont.

All of the major arteries leading to Fixx's heart were obstructed by arteriosclerosis, according to Eleanor N. McQuillen, Vermont's chief medical examiner, who autopsied Fixx. His left main coronary artery was almost completely blocked and his right one was 80 percent blocked. Even the arteries in his legs had blockages, McQuillen reported. Immediately, the Bassler hypothesis was held up to ridicule. Wasn't Fixx's death, at age 52, proof of how wrong he was, skeptics asked.

Some rushed to defend exercise against the onslaught of doubters and scoffers. A month after Fixx's death, novelist James A. Michener wrote: "The dramatic death of James F. Fixx, guru of exercise fanatics, of whom I am one, has thrown a scare into the jogging community." He recalled a conversation he had had with President Dwight Eisenhower's doctor, Paul Dudley White. White had told Michener about eight factors that could predict heart attack risk. And Michener, ticking the factors off, decided that Fixx had been due for a heart attack anyway. Fixx's father had had a major heart attack at thirty-five and died of a heart attack at age forty-three. Before he started running, Fixx had been sixty-one pounds overweight and was smoking two packs of cigarettes a day. He also had high blood pressure. "Indeed, looking at his profile, one is surprised he lived to 40," Michener writes, concluding that "running did not shorten Mr. Fixx's life. It prolonged it by 15 years."

Did it make any sense to insist that running prolongs life, asked Henry A. Solomon, a New York cardiologist. Solomon, in his 1984 book *The Exercise Myth*, set out to debunk those studies that concluded that exercise helps the heart or that it prevents heart disease or that it extends life.

"Longevity is the most compelling of the promised protections of exercise," Solomon wrote. "Millions of today's exercise enthusiasts, seduced into the latest warm-up gear, designer labels sticking to their sweaty bodies, run, dance, stretch, and strain in the hope and expectation of living longer lives."

He argued that exercise proponents had seized on physiological changes that can take place with exercise—a slower resting heart rate, a faster return to a resting heart rate after exertion—and interpreted them as clear indications of better health. "No one has shown any biological advantage to a slower heartbeat," he insisted. "I have patients in their eighties and nineties who have somewhat rapid heartbeats and have had them since their childhoods," but that doesn't seem to have made them less healthy. "People with even severe coronary heart disease can be 'trained' with exercise, but it doesn't alter the fact or severity of their coronary artery disease." In fact, he asserted, the training effect does not even involve their heart—their muscles become more efficient in extracting oxygen from blood. Exercise training, Solomon insisted, is not going to stave off the effects of heart disease.

Cooper was outraged. He debated Solomon on the television show *Nightline*. The two argued about the safety of exercise. "He said I couldn't interpret my own statistics, quote unquote," Cooper recalls. "He said there's nothing objective that exercise does."

Those who wanted to hear that exercise was not a panacea continued to cite Fixx's death, with decided satisfaction. Sports columnist Robert Lipsyte reported in 1986 that on a visit to an indoor track where he customarily ran, he noticed a new sign. "It read, 'Don't Give These Signals a Second Thought. Act Immediately.' The sign went on to list the symptoms of a heart attack." Lipsyte was disturbed. How inappropriate, he thought. "I had seen an identical sign before, on the refrigerator door of a sedentary writer. That was troubling, but appropriate. But not here. Would you hang a sign on the Fountain of Youth, 'Don't Drink the Water'?"

A few years later, research studies began pointing to another conclusion: that perhaps the health benefits of exercise emerge from the most modest of efforts, that there is no need to run a marathon if you want to improve your health. Walking would suffice. This, for me, is the most surprising part of the story of exercise and health. It led to the admonitions to the public to get moderate exercise, advice that so often is interpreted to mean that moderate exercise will help you lose weight. But, no, I discover, it is all about the heart.

Among the first to supply evidence that convinced most medical and public-health researchers was Steve Blair. No one was more astonished by his results than he. Blair, like other exercise physiologists, had thought that it had been well established that those who exercise more and more vigorously are fitter, and that being fitter translates into being healthier and living longer. It was stunning to find that that notion was wrong.

Blair reported his results in 1989 in a paper published in the *Journal of the American Medical Association.* His study involved a group of healthy adults—10,224 men and 3,120 women—who had come to his institute for a medical exam that included a treadmill test to assess their physical fitness. The investigators tracked the health of these people for eight years, collecting data that might allow them to associate any particular factors, like cholesterol levels or blood pressure or fitness, with an increased risk of death. They found that the greatest gains in fitness and longevity and health come from exercising enough so that you move out of the lowest quintile of fitness, basically the group that is completely sedentary, and into the second-lowest quintile of fitness.

In his paper, Blair was careful to note the study's limitations— and he said in interviews that he is well aware that he can never entirely discount the greatest limitation of all: The only way to be sure a study's participants are healthier because they exercise, not that they exercise because they are healthier, would be to do a very different study from his. Scientists would have to randomly assign thousands of people to exercise or not, and then to follow them for years, maybe even decades, to see if exercise made a difference to health. Such a study cannot be done, Blair insists, because it would cost billions and no one knows how to get a group of people to exercise for years on end. Moreover, he, for one, would find it unethical to assign half the subjects to be sedentary, for purposes of comparison. So, with that caveat, Blair must make the best of the study he has, pointing out that the study participants were not typical Americans: more than 99 percent were white, most were professionals, and most were college graduates. In addition, as is expected in such research, the investigators had to rely on statistical modeling to analyze the 283 deaths in the study, reporting the mortality rates in terms of "age-adjusted rates per 10,000 person-years."

Their daunting task was to account mathematically for the inherent differences between the participants in the different fitness groups. They took into account the factors like differences in age, in likelihood of being overweight, in blood pressure, cholesterol levels, and smoking history. But what if the people who were more physically fit just happened to be that way, not necessarily because they exercised more but simply because their bodies were healthier? Impossible to prove wrong but, in his opinion, not likely, Blair says. In general, fitness is a sign that someone exercises. In fact, he said, it probably is more accurate to measure physical activity by measuring physical fitness than by simply asking people how much they exercise.

"Moderate levels of physical fitness that are attainable by most adults appear to be protective against early mortality," the group wrote in its paper.

Women and men respond in the same way, other studies found. For example, a study by JoAnn E. Manson and her colleagues at Harvard Medical School published in 1999 in the *New England Journal of Medicine* involved 72,488 female nurses who were between the ages of forty and sixty-five when the study began. Over the next eight years, the researchers kept track of heart attacks and deaths from heart disease among the women, and sought to determine if those who exercised had less heart disease.

They reported that women who walked for three or more

hours a week had a 30 to 40 percent lower risk of heart disease as compared to more sedentary women and that such a moderate amount of exercise was sufficient—women who exercised more vigorously did not enjoy greater risk reductions.

And it does not matter if that mild exercise is done in a few long sessions or in numerous shorter ones, scientists reported. That, for example, was the conclusion drawn by Ralph S. Paffenbarger of Stanford University, who looked at exercise and heart disease among 7,307 male Harvard alumni. His data indicate that all that mattered was the total expenditure of energy. "Even men who only walked and climbed stairs and did not report additional participation in sports or recreational activities fared as well as those who engaged in sports or recreational activities, provided their total energy output was similar," he wrote in the journal *Circulation.*

"If you look at the lowest quintile of fitness, those are the people who account for the bulk of the mortality risk," says Michael Lauer, a cardiologist and research director at the Cleveland Clinic. "The mortality difference between average fitness and good and excellent fitness is really very small."

Blair looked back at the old studies he and others had relied on and asked why he and virtually everyone else in the exercise field had been misled into thinking that the more vigorous the exercise, the better. He found the studies that purported to demonstrate health benefits were actually looking at training effects—how the body responds to exertion. It was assumed that the better the response, the healthier the person was. Even so, those studies are almost laughable by today's standards. Their subjects were not randomly selected (nor were they even particularly representative of any broad group of people). And they involved so few subjects that it is hard to see how they could have reached reasonable conclusions.

One of the first of these studies, by a leading Finnish physiologist, Martti Karvonen, was published in 1957. Blair said he considers it "a classic" because it was one of the first controlled studies of exercise training.

Karvonen, who was Surgeon General of the Finnish army and founder and the first director of the Finnish Occupational Health Institute, is a towering figure in medicine, famous for his role in organizing and helping to lead a landmark study of heart disease. Known as the Seven Countries Study, it lasted from the mid-1950s until 1970 and compared disease and diet in seven countries, including Finland. Its findings helped launch the hypothesis that people who ate high-fat diets were more likely to develop heart disease.

His exercise training study is another matter. Blair says it should be looked at in the context of its time, as one of the first attempts to ask whether training made a difference in fitness. Karvonen concluded that it did, and his paper had a profound impact for decades to come.

Yet it involved just six young men, college students ages twenty to twenty-three. In the four-week-long experiment, the students ran on a treadmill for thirty minutes a day four or five days a week. Three kept their heart rates at 60 percent of their maximum and three kept their heart rates at 71 to 75 percent of their maximum, and one young man repeated the experiment, giving Karvonen and his colleagues a total of seven data points. The researchers reported that the students who trained at the higher heart rates got more fit—they ran faster at the end of the training period—and that those who trained less intensely did not improve.

After the Karvonen study, other investigators did similar experiments, with similar flaws. One, a 1967 study by Brian J. Sharkey, an exercise physiologist from the University of Montana in Missoula, published in 1967 in *Medicine and Science in Sports*, involved sixteen college men who exercised in sixteen sessions with ten-minute walks on a treadmill at different intensities. Another, conducted in 1970 by Irvin Faria of California State University in Sacramento, and published in *Research Quarterly for Exercise and Sport*, was a month-long study of forty college men divided into four groups who exercised five days a week by stepping on and off a bench.

Researchers evaluating clinical studies usually ask for tests of statistical significance, an assessment of whether the results are likely to have occurred simply by chance and not because there was a real physiological effect. But studies with statistically significant results must have enough people in them for the statistical tests to be valid. It would not be surprising if a coin happens to turn up heads three times out of four, but if it turns up heads 300 times out of 400 you would suspect some outside force was at work.

Reviewing the early exercise studies, Blair writes, "Lack of statistically significant findings for some of the studies is not surprising, given the low statistical power resulting from the small sample size (the largest group sampled was greater than ten in one study and less than ten in all others.)" Blair also notes that almost all of the studies that established the exercise dogma involved young men who were already fit. "The question being asked was, is high intensity exercise better than moderate? not, is moderate exercise also good?" Blair explained. That, of course, was the wrong question because it guaranteed that the large health effect of going from no exercise to some exercise would be missed. The questions that are most important to public-health specialists are very different: What happens when a middle-aged or older person who is completely sedentary starts a modest exercise program? Can exercise help even people who already have heart disease? Large studies, like Blair's, indicate that even modest efforts can improve health.

For Blair, his 1989 study was enough. He immediately revised his message and his focus. Almost overnight, the emphasis of most exercise physiologists changed. Instead of studying intense exercise and how to train most effectively, the focus became: How little can you do and still get a health benefit? The amount of recommended exercise dropped, and dropped again. First it was a half-hour walk a day five days a week, or something equally mild, like an easy bike ride. Then it was to walk twenty minutes a day five days a week. Then it was get in twenty to thirty minutes of walking—and not necessarily consecutive minutes—at least three days a week. The minutes count even if you do something as simple as walk from the outer edge of a parking lot to your office.

The challenge, notes Lauer, the Cleveland Clinic cardiologist, is to encourage people to exercise without frightening them off with activities that seem much too hard. If sedentary people think their goal is the kind of maximum-heart-rate, all-out push that the people in my Spinning classes want, "a lot of people would be so daunted that they wouldn't even try," he says.

As Lauer points out, "My parents always wanted me to be above average, but this is one area where average is fine."

Even Cooper changed his message. He no longer insists that you have to be aerobically fit, according to his test and point system, to stay healthy. All you need, he agrees, is moderate exercise, a two-mile walk accomplished in thirty minutes three times a week, or two miles in forty minutes five times a week. The real problem, he says, is with the huge number of people who do not exercise at all.

"At least forty-nine million [American] adults are totally sedentary," Cooper asserts. "That's a deplorable thing. And the majority are there because they want to be there. They just have a poor attitude toward fitness and health. They are lackadaisical. They always have excuses."

"This is a very important message," Lauer stresses, and especially so for the heart-disease patients he so often sees. "Cardiac patients by their very nature tend to be sedentary. It's important to tell them you don't have to be a marathon runner. What we are asking for is really very mild levels of activity, but they need to occur pretty often, thirty minutes a day for at least three days a week."

To me, this sounds like exercise as medicine. If someone told me to go for a ten-minute walk three times a day I'd think of it as an obligation on the order of taking a pill three times a day. I certainly wouldn't expect to look any better. For sure, I wouldn't lose any weight. Wouldn't it be more fun to exercise a little more intensely?

That brings me back to the fundamental question: Why exercise? Despite the constant exhortations to the American public, dating back to the Eisenhower era, the public-health push to get people to exercise has been pretty much a failure. Most Americans ignored the advice in the days when exercise physiologists said more is better. And when they switched to saying that all you need is the most minimal of movement, the advice was, if anything, ignored even more roundly by the majority of the public. For decades now, the Centers for Disease Control and Prevention has kept track of the nation's exercise habits through its National Health and Nutrition Surveys. And it finds that now, as in previous years, as much as 60 percent of the population gets no regular exercise.

At the same time, many of those who have always exercised continued to do so, at their old pace, even as the public-health message changed, telling them they did not have to do so much. The regulars at Gold's Gym say they are not thinking about their hearts as they push their bodies. Joe Alfano, a young stock trader, exercises because it makes him feel so good—exhilarated, vigorous, melting away the stress of his job, at least for the moment. He loves that feeling so much that he cannot stay away from the gym for more than a few days, even though getting there requires careful attention to his schedule and, often, rushing away from work as the day draws to a close. What about his health, his heart, I ask him? That, he tells me, is not the reason he works out.

"Why do *you* work out?" Joe asks me. For the same reasons he does, I reply. And the more hours I spend at my job, the more

I crave a vigorous exercise session. The second week of July 2002 was the perfect example. It was an unusual week, with several major news stories that I had to cover, and I was finding it impossible to get away.

On Monday, July 9, I was at my desk in New York at eight-thirty in the morning and did not get home until ten that night—too late to exercise. The gyms in my town close at 10:00 p.m., and it was hot and muggy outside, not the kind of evening that tempted me to go for a run in the dark. Anyway, I had not yet had dinner.

The next day I worked at home, but the day lasted fourteen hours and, once again, there was no chance to get away. Wednesday, I worked at home again, starting at 7:00 a.m. and finally ending at 6:30 p.m. All day, I had been feeling tired, dragged down by the intense effort and pressure of the job. When I saw an opportunity to leave my work for a couple of hours, I dashed to Gold's Gym in time for the 7:00 p.m. Spinning class. I pushed myself hard and by the time it was over, I felt renewed, totally invigorated, euphoric. I knew, once again, why I love exercise.

I ask Steve Blair if he has changed his own exercise habits and he says no, he has not. He still runs every day, and he still runs marathons. "It's part of who I am," he tells me. He adds that he enjoys running, that it helps clear his mind, and the intense exercise also helps him control his weight—not to be thin, he says, but to be *thinner* than he would be if he did not run each day.

"I was short, fat, and bald when I started running, and I'm still short, fat, and bald. Weight control is difficult for me—I fight the losing battle. I've run seventy-five thousand miles and gained twenty pounds in the last thirty-five years." He says there is a limit to what exercise can do to keep his weight down. "It's much easier to eat a thousand calories than to burn a thousand calories," Blair says. "An old football coach used to say, 'I have all my assistants running five miles a day, but they eat ten miles a day.' " Nonetheless, Blair confirms, "being physically active tends to make you weigh less. That's not to say that everyone who is highly active is skinny, just as it's not to say that everyone who is skinny is highly active."

I ask others what drives them to exercise vigorously and often, and the answers are almost always the same: weight control; a sense of power, and even superiority; pride in the way their bodies look and perform; the exhilaration of a hard workout; stress relief. Few tell me they are doing it for their health or to reduce their chances of dying in the next few years.

"The pure and simple reason why we exercise year after year is that it makes you feel good," Cooper admitted. "People who are physically fit are less depressed, they have less hypochondria, they are different psychologically." Hundreds—thousands—of people have given him that reason, and it is the reason why Cooper himself exercises, he says. "I challenge people all the time. 'You think you feel good now? Try exercising.' "

Dan Zwick, a computer scientist living in Germany and a marathon runner, wrote to me after reading one of my *New York Times* articles on exercise. He told me that he lost more than thirty pounds when he became a marathon runner, and, just as important, he said, he gained a new persona.

"When things seemed unbearable in my life, I told myself: You're a marathon runner—you've withstood worse pain than this! But it also worked the other way. During a temporary weak spell in the Boston Marathon, I told myself: You've been through hell; you can get through this, too!"

Even Dave Costill, an august exercise physiologist from Ball State University, now semiretired, is not immune to the vanity factor. Tall and lean, with an athlete's easy grace, at age sixty-five he still swims each day with much younger men and competes against others in his age group, clocking times as fast as when he was in college. He also runs. When I ask Costill why he exercises, he says it is in part because he likes the discipline and the self-image it gives him, training even on days when he does not really want to. "For me it's a certain satisfaction of personal maintenance," Costill says. "I feel like exercise is an important part of my life, and if I don't do it, I'm just being lazy. A lot of people exercise for health, but that's not me. I ask myself, 'Is this as good as my body is capable of being?' "

He runs, he says, partly to control his weight. Although he looks naturally thin, even he worries about extra pounds creeping on.

Still, fears of intense exercise linger.

I wonder how many people are afraid to exercise because they worry about their hearts—not people who had heart attacks but people who have heart murmurs or irregular rhythms or enlarged hearts. If I had had different doctors, would I be one of them?

I had always assumed that my heart was fine until I was hired by the *New York Times* in 1987 and went to the *Times*'s medical office on the fifth floor of the building to have the required tests, which included an electrocardiogram. I had never had one before and was astonished when the nurse doing the test advised me to see a cardiologist because my results were abnormal. I put it off, worried about getting caught in the maws of the medical-testing maze like my friend Denise, who told me about how she had undergone test after sophisticated test for her heart only to be told in the end that nothing serious was wrong. She was relieved, in a way, but resented the hundreds of dollars and countless hours it cost her to find out.

About a decade later, when I had a routine checkup, my doctor did an electrocardiogram. She informed me that it was abnormal but she was not worried about it because she thought it was a result of all the exercise I do. She did, however, hear a murmur in my heart and sent me on for an echocardiogram ($650). "Clinically insignificant," the results came back.

And then there is my slow heart beat, slow enough to be called bradycardia, a resting heart beat below sixty beats per minute. Cardiologist Paul Thompson says that such a slow heart rate can be a sign of heart disease. It also can be a sign that you exercise a lot.

Despite the ever-increasing body of evidence that the murmurs, irregular heart beats, slow resting heart rates, and enlarged hearts they see in athletes are healthy and normal adaptations to exercise, some doctors worry. "There's still a lot of debate about it," Thompson says. Even now, in the July 2002 issue of *Physician and Sportsmedicine*, a journal for practicing doctors, the issue of athlete's heart crops up.

In an article titled "The Athletic Heart Syndrome: Ruling Out Cardiac Pathologies," James C. Puffer, professor and chief of sports medicine at the University of California, Los Angeles, advises doctors that athletes often have hearts that might look abnormal but that the abnormality is generally a response to training, not a sign of disease. He details how to evaluate athletes and concludes: "Few things can be more alarming than concerns about underlying cardiac disease. Thus, when evaluation reveals no evidence of significant disease, the clinician must place this in proper context. Reassurance that such findings are a normal response to training will allow the athlete to return to full activity without worrying that 'something may be wrong with my heart.' "

four

MAXIMUM HEART RATES
AND FAT-BURNING ZONES

I have become an acute observer of my heart. I know how fast it beats when I am standing around at the gym. I know how fast it beats when I exercise hard enough to be out of breath. I know its maximum rate and I know how quickly that falls when I stop exercising.

My almost obsessive fascination with monitoring my heart began not because I thought there was anything wrong with it but because I discovered Spinning. It is a sport that has led me into a world of heart-rate training that I barely knew existed. It is a world that uses the heart as a way to assess the body and the effects of exercise, and raises questions such as: Where do the formulas for calculating your maximum heart rate come from? Can they be trusted? And: Is there a special "fat-burning zone" where your heart is beating at just the right rate so you burn the most fat possible when you exercise?

But those questions were farthest from my mind on the cold evening in November of 2000 when I first stepped into a Spinning room. I was there to accompany my husband, Bill, who had decided that Spinning might be a solution to his annual funk. Bill only likes one type of exercise—bicycling; and only one type of bicycling—road riding, as opposed to mountain biking. Every year, the pattern is the same. In September, when it gets dark so early that he can't ride his bike after work, he starts to feel downcast. By January, when it gets truly cold and the roads get so slushy or icy that he no longer wants to ride outside even on weekends, he gets even more discouraged. While others might say they feel glum because it's winter, with its short days that force you to go to work in the darkness and return home after the sun sets, Bill attributes his gray moods to an inability to exercise the way he wants to. For months on end, he is relegated to riding stationary bikes at the gym. And, as he is quick to tell me, those computer-controlled exercise machines are not only boring but they do not look or feel like a real road bike.

That year, Bill decides he wants to try something new. He's been noticing the Spinning classes in a little glass-walled area just behind the treadmills at our gym. There, in a darkened room, on stationary bikes that look remotely like road bikes, he sees sweaty people pedaling away to music, led by an instructor at the front of the room. It is hard to tell just what is going on, since the instructor always turns off the lights when the class starts, but the class seems to do more than simply sit back and pedal their bikes. They also rise from their seats to stand straight up, and sometimes to pedal leaning forward over the handlebars. The only alternative being a LifeCycle, Bill reasons, what does he have to lose?

At the very least curious, I join him, and we arrive with our mandatory water bottles and sweat towels. We are also wearing special bicycling shoes, which clip directly to the pedals to afford us the most efficient motion—as your foot rises, your shoe pulls the pedal up. We are ready to learn the mechanics of Spinning.

The bikes are set in sturdy metal frames, and have only one wheel, a heavy metal flywheel, in front. But that's okay, because you're not going anywhere on these bikes. You adjust the seat's height by moving it up or down on a post, and you adjust its distance from the handlebars by sliding it forward or backward along a metal bar. The handlebars point forward like a bull's horns, and you can move them higher or lower. The seat is narrow and hard, like the seat on a racing bike. There is a cage on the bike frame, in front of and below the seat, where you can slip a plastic bottle of water. There also is a round knob on the frame, just below the fork that holds the front wheel, that you can turn to increase or decrease the resistance on the pedals. The way it works is when you turn the knob for more resistance, on either side of the front wheel, pads close in, pressing against the wheel with variable pressure. The pads, about three inches long and about an inch and a half wide, are made of fiber that has the texture of industrial carpeting. They slow the wheel by friction as they push against it, and the more you turn the resistance knob, the harder they press against the wheel. Your job is to overcome the force of friction that they generate. It is like trying to ride a bike with the brake on; the harder you push on the brake, the harder you will have to pedal to turn the wheel.

You set up your bike so it fits you. The seat must be high enough so that when you extend your leg, with your foot on the pedal, your leg should be extended, but not so much that your knee is locked. The angle between the upper part of your leg and the lower part of your leg should be about twenty degrees. Your handlebars can be one or two inches above or below your seat, depending on your preference. When you reach out for the handlebars, your arms should be extended but your elbows must not be locked.

In class, you sit, stand, or lean forward on your bike, pedaling in time to the music. You turn the knob that increases or decreases the resistance while you simulate climbing a hill or sprinting on a flat stretch of road—or, sometimes, sprinting up a hill. If you put your mind to it, turning the resistance knob enough and pedaling fast enough so that you are exerting real effort, you can get a hard, heart-pounding workout, we discover. It can be as difficult as a fast run; and, I learn, it can make me feel as good.

So, to our great surprise, Bill and I become Spinning enthusiasts, taking the forty-minute classes two, three, even four nights a week. Sometimes, we find ourselves setting an alarm and waking up early on Saturday mornings to take Spinning classes. At our gym, those weekend classes are crowded, and because some bikes are better than others, the only way to be sure you have the best Spinning experience is to come an hour or so before class and drape your towel over the bike you want. While you wait for the class to begin, you lift weights.

One Thursday night, after we've been taking Spinning classes for a few weeks, Anna Hess, the instructor, takes me aside. This warm blonde is also a personal trainer and a marathon runner, and it shows. A short and compact powerhouse, Anna seems driven to inspire the class to take Spinning seriously, not just pedaling along at a low resistance, as most people seem to do, but working at a precisely measured pace. She has us tap our knee with each pedal stroke and count how many times per minute we turn the pedals, making sure we keep up our cadence. She admonishes us to keep track of our heart rates, if not with a heart-rate monitor, then by putting a finger to the carotid artery in our necks and counting our pulse.

Anna wanted to tell me about a special Spinning class that is being planned at another gym where she also teaches. It is going to be a four-hour Spinning climb, called Mount Everest, and we can sign up for it if we want to, training at our gym and the gym where the ride will take place. Are we interested?

Bill demurs, wondering how much time and effort he really wants to devote to this indoor sport and wondering why anyone would want to spend four hours in a hot little room, on a Spinning bike, with the resistance turned up, simulating a climb. I, however, am all for it. How could we not do it, I ask Bill. I think of it as a form of Extreme Spinning and decide that it will be, at the very least, memorable. It will also be an opportunity to test our physical limits. I remember what my son, Stefan, says about my running programs. "The way you run is so boring," he tells me. "It's like you're always between seasons, never training for anything." This is our chance to see if we can go from forty-minute classes to a four-hour climb.

We sign up for the class. We have about two months to train.

The first thing we have to do, Anna tells us, is get heart-rate monitors. They are mandatory for the Mount Everest ride. I'd always questioned why I would want one. To use it, you strap an elastic band around your chest. In front is a plastic strip with two flat sections that you wet with water so they maintain a tight contact with your chest. They contain sensors that pick up your heart's electrical signals, convert them into radiowave signals, and transmit them to a device that looks like a wristwatch that displays the data in terms of heart beats per minute. I've seen them on men who are running shirtless. They had seemed absurd to me—with this wide strap across their chests, like a sort of mini-bra. I wondered where a woman would put the strap. Across her breasts? I could not imagine it. But it turns out that you can put the strap just below your bra. It began to seem a little less weird, although still definitely a bit extreme.

Now that I'm taking Spinning classes, however, I can see why heart-rate monitors make sense. If you want to improve—and that, after all, is the point of training—you have to have some way of assessing your performance objectively. If you run, you can get a pretty good idea of what kind of a workout you did—you can see how far you ran and how long it took you. But Spinning is so abstract, it offers no such gauge. You cannot even try to guess at your effort by how hard you are breathing—the music is so loud, you cannot hear yourself breathe. And you can't tell how hard you are working by how hot you become because the temperature can vary in the little room, and you may or may not be near a fan to cool yourself.

What you want to know is your effort, your watts, a unit of power that is the equivalent of calories burned over time. Spinning bikes are not designed with wattmeters, so you are left with two indirect measures of your effort. One is your cadence, how quickly you are pushing the pedals. If you keep the resistance constant, the faster you move the pedals, the harder you are working. There is, however, a problem with using cadence, and it is one that shows up in every Spinning class I've ever been in. I see people who are pedaling away, at astonishing rates, but with virtually no resistance on their flywheels. Once you start pedaling with the resistance knob turned to zero, the heavy wheel will turn fast on its own, from its own momentum. Although your pedals are whirling, you are essentially just going along for the ride. You are putting out almost no effort, and burning almost no calories, even though it looks like you are blazing along at an impressive speed.

That leaves heart rate as a measure of effort. It is an indirect indicator, because although your heart beats faster and faster as your effort gets greater and greater, the relationship is linear only at the lower levels of effort. As your effort increases, the heart rate creeps toward a plateau, your maximum heart rate. That means you can increase your effort, burning more calories, and see only a tiny change in how quickly your heart is beating. It is a bit frustrating—the harder you work, the less effect you see in your heart rate—and when you are working hardest, you'd like to be rewarded with a real rise in your beats per minute. But with this limitation: the higher your heart rate, the more calories you are burning and the harder you are working.

The physics is straightforward, although the interpretation of heart rates, I soon discover, is mired in myths and misconceptions, in pseudo-science and marketing. It starts with the charts that show up in every gym, supplied by any of a variety of companies. They give the maximum number of heartbeats per minute for someone your age and specify the training value of different percentages of that rate. An instructor may tell you to get your heart rate up to 65 percent of your maximum as you warm up and then to get it to 80 percent as you increase your resistance for the first "hill." That sort of advice only makes sense if you have a heart-rate monitor, of course. Who knows what it feels like to work at 80 percent of your maximum heart rate? Even checking your pulse by putting a finger on your neck can be misleading. You can only check when you take a break, and your heart rate should start plummeting the moment you ease off on your pedaling. As Bill and I discovered when we compared ten-second pulse checks to the heart-rate monitor readings, the pulse checks can be wildly inaccurate.

So we get our monitors, put them on, peruse the chart to see what our maximum heart rates should be, and take a Spinning class. We do not question the figures on the chart, and we assume that those figures—65 percent of maximum, 80 percent of maximum—mean something. We just look at what the chart says should be our heart rates and decide that those will be our goals.

Immediately, something seems wrong. If I exercise so that my monitor displays heart rates like the ones the chart says are my goals, I feel like I'm barely moving. I find that if I am at 80 percent of what, according to my age, should be my maximum, it is as if I am coasting along. Yet 80 percent marks what is supposed to be a transition, where you are starting to sweat and breathe hard, where you should find it hard to carry on a conversation. If, however, I work as hard as I think I should, pushing myself until I really am sweating and breathing hard, my heart rate is off the chart. Where, I wonder, did these rates come from? Does anyone trust them?

"That formula is for babies," one woman at my gym scornfully informs me. Her theory is that it purposely gives heart rates that are too low so that nonathletes trying to use exercise equipment won't get injured. I decide to investigate. Soon, I learn that most standard charts are based on a simple formula: your maximum heart rate equals 220 minus your age. Your maximum heart rate is the fastest your heart can beat, and when you get even close to that rate, you enter into a so-called anaerobic zone, which is so hard to maintain that you can only keep it up for a few minutes. Your anaerobic zone is about 90 to 95 percent of your maximum heart rate.

Those charts, that formula, I find, are everywhere—they are by no means something that was devised for Spinning. The heart-rate charts are even in medical textbooks and in doctors' offices. If you go in for a treadmill test to see if you have signs of heart disease, your doctor will ask you to start walking on a treadmill while the speed and incline gradually are increased. All the while, the doctor will be monitoring your heart rate, stopping the test when you reach 80 percent of your maximum, according to a chart based on the same 220-minus-your-age formula.

Doctors I asked seemed never to have questioned the charts. One leading cardiologist, Steve Nissen, at the Cleveland Clinic, solemnly assured me that the formula is correct. "It is based on real data," he said.

Some athletes, notably Lance Armstrong, the champion cyclist who came back from testicular cancer to win the hardest bicycle race in the world, the Tour de France, are avid promoters of monitoring their heart rates while they exercise. "Lance is never far from his heart-rate monitor—he wears it on 90 percent of his rides," his coach, Chris Carmichael, writes.

The standard formula is programmed into exercise machines. There are variations of it—the "fat-burning zone," which is about 50 to 60 percent of your maximum heart rate; the "training zone," at about 75 to 85 percent. My current favorite machine, a popular model of the elliptical trainer, can display your heart rate and show you whether, according to its formula, it is at an appropriate level. The machine's display panel has a little horizontal gauge like a thermometer's with a scale that goes from the slowest heart rate to the fastest, from red ("below zone") to yellow ("weight loss") to green ("cardiovascular") to another red area—the "above zone." Now I understand it.

But the more I saw of that heart-rate formula, the more I wondered about it, whether in Spinning classes or on the elliptical trainer or even exercising outdoors. In theory, if you exercise "above zone," in your anaerobic range, you should be panting for breath, feeling like you are in an all-out sprint. Even thirty seconds of effort at that pace should be very hard.

I step on the elliptical trainer and start entering the parameters for my exercise session—duration, level, the pattern of hills and valleys. As always, the machine asks my age. I always just punch "Enter" at that question, rather than moving an arrow to the right age. So, invariably, the machine thinks I am thirty-five, its default age. As I start the exercise session, I watch my heart rate, and I watch the gauge that interprets it for me. In seconds, I have moved into the "weight-loss zone," a heart rate so low that I cannot conceive of exercising at that level. Soon, I am moving into the "cardiovascular zone"; once again, not much of an effort until I get near the top of the zone (for a thirty-five-year-old), where the effort feels about right, at around 155 beats per minute. I keep going, though, and soon I am in the red area of the heart-rate gauge—"above zone"— something that happens on this machine as soon as I surpass 157 beats per minute, which the machine thinks is 85 percent of a thirty-five-year-old's maximum of 185 beats per minute. I'm exercising vigorously, breathing hard and sweating, but it is not so hard that I cannot keep going, and I remain in that red zone for about 40 minutes. I have even had my average heart rate—which includes the 5 minutes or so it can take to warm up and really get going—be as high as 159 beats a minute for a 40- to 45-minute workout.

If the formula was right, that should have been anaerobic exercise for someone younger than I, whose heart rate should be faster than mine. It should be impossible to stay in the red zone for more than a few minutes. Granted, it was a hard workout; but if red meant anaerobic, I must be a physiological freak.

How seriously do exercise physiologists take this formula? And where did it come from?

Donald Kirkendall, an exercise physiologist at the University of North Carolina, will never forget the time he put a heart-rate

monitor on a member of the United States rowing team and asked
the man to row as hard as he could for six minutes. The man was
in his early twenties, and so his maximum heart rate should be
somewhere below 200—and no one can maintain a heart rate at
its maximum level for long.

"His pulse rate hit two hundred at ninety seconds into the
test," Kirkendall says. "And he held it there for the rest of the
test. A local cardiologist was looking on in astonishment. He
said, 'You know, there's not a textbook in the world that says a
person could have done that.' " Another time, he put a heart-rate
monitor on a young woman playing a championship soccer
match. Her average heart rate for the two hours of play was
190—a physiological impossibility if the formula was correct.

Fritz Hagerman, an exercise physiologist at Ohio University
and an expert on champion rowers, has also seen athletes whose
heart rates are stratospheric. But a high heart rate does not mean
an athlete is particularly talented. The reason your heart speeds
up when you exercise is that your muscles are crying out for
blood. There are two ways to get blood to your muscles: your
heart can pump more blood with each beat or your heart can beat
faster. Each person uses a different combination of these functions, Hagerman says, something he realized when he studied
champion rowers.

"You can start off with two people in a boat and ask them to
go two thousand meters," Hagerman told me. "You may have
one athlete who has great muscles for soaking up oxygen—he can
soak it up like crazy. Part of that is inherited and part comes from
training. The other athlete doesn't have that kind of muscle fiber,
but he has this huge heart that can deliver a lot of blood. One
athlete gets oxygen to his muscles by transport, pumping blood
fast, and the other gets it there by pumping a lot of blood with
each beat and soaking up all the oxygen in it."

He says he can be working with two Olympic rowers, equally
able to perform. The one whose body's strategy is to pump blood
fast will have a maximum heart rate of 220, and the other, whose

strategy is to pump a lot of blood with each beat, will have a maximum of 160. As a result, Hagerman does not pay much attention to maximum heart rates in the rowers he trains. "The heart rate is probably the least important variable in comparing athletes," he says.

Kirkendall also finds maximum heart rates uninformative when it comes to athletes, and he shares Hagerman's skepticism of the formula, even though it has been used uncritically ever since the exercise movement began in the early 1970s.

It originated in the late sixties when William Haskell, an exercise physiologist who is now at Stanford University, and Sam Fox, a cardiologist, provided a formula for maximum heart rates for people who were having treadmill stress tests for heart disease. Their paper, published in 1970 in a book, *Research Conference on Applied Work Physiology*, was not really a scientific effort; rather, it was a suggestion, based on a decidedly nonrandom and small sample of people, that the 220-minus-age formula might best fit the data points. Haskell is a sophisticated and highly regarded scientist, not one with a reputation for misrepresenting data. So I ask him to tell me his story.

It was 1968, Haskell said, and he had recently gotten his Ph.D. in exercise physiology and was employed by the U.S. Public Health Service, one of thousands of doctors and scientists who work in government offices and laboratories under the direction of the Surgeon General. His job put him under the supervision of Sam Fox, a doctor who was the head of a major heart-disease prevention program in the Public Health Service. It was a time when heart-attack patients were first being encouraged to exercise, and when both doctors and patients were a bit nervous about the exercise prescription. How could people with heart disease judge when they were exercising enough to help their hearts and how could they know when to cut back because they might be exercising so vigorously that they could be in danger of a new heart attack?

One idea was to see whether people's heart rates could be used to estimate exercise intensity. Fox had been invited to give a talk at a World Health Organization meeting on the use of exercise testing to detect heart disease, and so he asked Haskell to help him prepare, sending him to the library to gather papers in which people of different ages had been tested to find their maximum heart rates. Haskell found seven papers and plotted the data on a piece of graph paper.

Shortly afterward, Haskell and Fox were on their way to another meeting—Haskell no longer remembers where they were going, explaining that they traveled a lot in those days. But he does vividly recall what happened while they were sitting together on a long airplane ride. Haskell pulled out his plot and showed it to Fox. "We drew a line through it and I said 'Gee, if you extrapolate that out, it looks like at twenty, your maximum heart rate is two hundred, at age forty it's a hundred and eighty, at sixty it's one-sixty . . .'" Fox, he says, turned to him and said, "It looks like two-twenty minus your age."

The two presented the graph at another meeting, this time in Tel Aviv, publishing it in the conference's proceedings, which appeared as a book in 1970, *Cardiology: Current Topics and Progress*. At yet another meeting that year, held in Tuxedo Park, New York, they presented, for the first time, the mathematical equation, as opposed to just the graph, in the chapter of a book on the conference proceedings, *Research Conference on Applied Work Physiology*. Finally, in 1971, Fox and Haskell published a graph based on ten studies, rather than the original seven, along with their formula, concluding, once again, that the formula *maximum heart rate equals 220 minus age* best fit the data.

Most participants in those ten studies were under age sixty-five, and all were men. While those were the usual subjects in medical studies in those days, investigators today would ask whether the formula would hold for women or old people. Beyond that, however, was a broader question. Were the published data on maximum heart rates reliable? Scientists who set out to find people's maximum heart rates at different ages should, ideally, recruit random samples of healthy people in different age groups. It should be done like the sampling of the population in opinion polls—with groups that represent the population—men and, perhaps separately, women in each decade of adult life, for example. And each group should contain enough people for the scientists to have confidence that their findings are reliable. The investigators would measure each person's maximum heart rate, determining, in the end, not just what the average maximum heart rate is at different ages, but how much an individual's rate might vary, up or down, from the average figures.

Instead, the investigators who published those heart-rate studies used what scientists call samples of convenience. Or, as Kirkendall puts it, "pretty much anyone who came in the door." That, of course, introduces biases. Who would walk in the door? People who had heart disease and were worried about exercising? Athletes who wanted to test their limits? It is easy to end up with a group that does not at all resemble the norm. But, Kirkendall remarks, "in the exercise field, a true random sample is pretty rare."

There's another problem, too. Imagine someone who has never exercised taking a treadmill test. They will be asked to walk faster and faster on a treadmill slope that is getting increasingly steeper. The test ends when they cannot continue. And their heart rate when the treadmill is stopped is supposed to be their maximum. But is it? It may well be, says Kirkendall, that it is not their hearts that are the limiting factor.

"From having done lots of exercise tests on people who don't exercise, I can tell you that as the hill gets steep, their calves will start complaining and they will say they can't go any farther. There's a possibility that you're not getting a maximum heart rate because they quit on you early," he says. "Most people have no idea how hard they can work."

Douglas Seals, an exercise physiologist at the University of Colorado, agrees. "For people who don't exercise vigorously, there's a huge error. They may not be anywhere close to their maximum and they tell you they are."

Haskell is aware of the limitations of the formula—a nonrandom sample of men, no real guarantee that any of them got to their maximum heart rate, extrapolations from younger ages to older ones. But, he says, the formula has been useful. One thing it showed was a new physical phenomenon—that the maximum heart rate slows by about a beat a year throughout adult life. No one has ever been able to figure out why, and many have tried, including Haskell himself.

The formula also has practical uses, Haskell says. He relies on it to help people decide how hard to exercise. "You tell them to exercise at a moderate intensity. Well, what's a moderate intensity? You say, 'Well, you're sweating.' And they say, "On a hot day I sweat anyway.' " How much easier to just point to the formula, pick out what is supposed to be 60 percent of the maximum heart rate, and tell the patients to wear a heart-rate monitor and get their heart rate to that level for twenty minutes several times a week.

Another advantage of the formula, Haskell says, is that it induces people to increase their effort gradually. As they get more fit, they will have to work harder and harder to get to their target heart rate. Those who are completely sedentary will find their heart rate soaring with minimal effort. They might run a block to catch a bus and find their heart pounding furiously for minutes after they board. A person who runs each day would hardly be winded by the same dash for a bus, and their heart rate would plummet as soon as they got on. As a sedentary person starts exercising, their body will adapt, so that what once was a hard workout becomes easy. And an effort that used to get their heart rate to a target zone is now insufficient. So, Haskell says, when he tells people to aim for a particular heart rate in each exercise session, "that automatically forces them to increase their workload as they get more fit."

Seals agrees. "There is a need, a clinical and societal need, to estimate the maximum heart rate." He is not wedded to Haskell's formula. "The more information we have, the more we realize that that formula is just a very rough consideration." Seals tried to improve the formula, gathering data from 351 published studies involving 18,712 people. To that he added his own data from studies involving 514 men and women, aged 18 to 81. Nearly half, 229 of them, had been doing exercises such as running or bicycling for at least two years and were trained for endurance. The remaining 285 were sedentary. None were smokers, none were obese, and none were taking drugs other than hormone replacement (taken by some of the postmenopausal women).

In Seals's studies, subjects walked or ran on a treadmill, at increasing speed and with an ever-increasing pitch to the treadmill's hill, until they could go no longer. Seals verified that they reached their maximum heart rates by looking for very rapid breathing, for oxygen consumption that had risen steadily and then leveled off because they could work no harder, and for the subjects' insistence that this was their maximum effort.

Seals reported that a person's maximum heart rate is independent of their physical fitness and their gender but does depend on how old they are. He concluded, in a paper published in the *American Journal of Cardiology* in 2001, that the traditional formula of 220 minus age overestimates the maximum rate in young adults, does a pretty good job for people who are around forty years old, and then increasingly underestimates the maximum rate as people get older. A much more accurate formula, he says, is 208 minus age times 0.7. Even with that formula individuals vary so much that someone's true maximum could be as much as twenty beats per minute higher or lower than the number the formula provides. But on average, he reported, his formula represents the data. Yet Seals, despite his impressive and exhaustive effort to get accurate data and derive a better formula, failed to supplant the old equation suggested by Haskell and Fox.

One reason for the persistence of the Haskell and Fox formula might be that not only is it enshrined in medical and physiology textbooks but it also became part of a business enterprise, a fact that, Haskell confesses ruefully, never occurred to him when he published the heart-rate equation.

The commercialization of the formula was first accomplished by a Finnish company, Polar Electro, which started making monitors in 1979, initially selling them to the Finnish Nordic Ski Team "to monitor the intensity of their workouts," as the company explains on its Web site. Now, Corey Cornaccio, the company's director of marketing in the United States, tells me, Americans buy more than three-quarters of a million heart-rate monitors each year. Most are sold to individuals who are not professional athletes but who use them to gauge their efforts when they work out. The company has an array of devices, increasingly elaborate and increasingly expensive. It even sells monitors for horses.

The variety of monitors seems limited only by the designers' imagination of what an exerciser might want to know. The simplest just displays your heart rate. That's the one I bought. From there on they get increasingly elaborate, beeping at you if you go above or below your target heart-rate zone, keeping track of time and distance, allowing you to recall what your heart rate was on previous workouts and to compare those rates with the ones on your current workout. The high-end monitor, the Polar Coach, costs about four times as much as the basic model and is geared to the truly obsessive. It tells you your heart rate, lap time, elapsed time, and time of day. It calculates the amount of time you spent in, above, and below your target heart-rate zone and calculates your average heart rate. It monitors how quickly your heart recovers from exercise by tracking the fall in the rate when you slow down, and it has a coded transmission of your heart rate so you avoid a problem that plagues some people in Spinning classes—accidentally getting your neighbor's heart rate displayed on your watch because you are picking up transmissions from the monitor strapped around your neighbor's chest. And just to be sure that no bit of information is lost, you can download data from the monitor to a computer.

Haskell is a bit taken aback by the way the heart-rate formula has come to be viewed almost as a physical law. "I've kind of laughed about it over the years," he says, adding, "It's typical of Americans to take an idea and extend it way beyond what it was intended for."

When he and Fox proposed the formula, they never intended to give an absolute number for athletes or people who are used to exercising vigorously. They never claimed to be providing a way to give a precise maximum heart rate for a given individual. In fact, it is clear from the widely scattered data points on the graphs of heart rates that any individual's maximum rate can vary widely from what that formula predicts, by as many as thirty beats per minute higher or lower. And that means that what you calculate as your training zone could be completely wrong. "If it says 150, it could be 180 or it could be 120," notes Jack Wilmore, an exercise physiologist at Texas A&M.

As anyone who has tried to measure their heart rate during exercise knows, those differences are huge. Most people would not find it hard to get their heart rate up to 120 beats a minute. Many would be walking briskly or jogging slowly and barely breaking a sweat. It's much harder to get your heart up to 150 beats a minute—you may have to run or even start to sprint. Reaching a heart rate of 180 requires substantial effort, running fast or running uphill, and many who try to reach that rate and sustain it will find that it is beyond their capacity.

If you want to train for an event, like the Mount Everest Spinning event, and if you misjudge your maximum heart rate, you can easily be thwarted. If I thought my maximum was 150 when it really was 180, I would hardly be exercising when I was supposed to be doing aerobic training at 80 percent of my maximum

heart rate. Eighty percent of 150 is 120; but 80 percent of 180 is
144—a huge difference in terms of effort.

It is clear from Seals's extensive work that there is no formula
to predict, ahead of time, precisely what a person's maximum
heart rate will be. But some of us are curious. I'd like to know
just how hard I can work, since I suspect that I could push myself
a lot harder. If I know my maximum heart rate, I may be able to
better gauge what I can do. The problem is that finding it can be
incredibly difficult if you try to do it on your own.

"This is not an easy test," writes Lance Armstrong's trainer,
Chris Carmichael. He recommends going harder and harder and
faster and faster on a bike, "until you simply can't go any harder."
Then, he says, "when your vision clears," look at your heart-rate
monitor. That should be your maximum.

John L. Parker, Jr., a runner, wrote about how to do it with
running. Start out on a day when you're well rested, he advises.
Warm up by running two to four miles at an easy pace. Then do
some sprints to get your heart rate up. Now you're ready for the
real event. You should start with a series of runs up a steep hill
about 200 to 300 yards long. Do it about five times, jogging
down then charging up, faster each time. On the last sprint up
that hill, "keep increasing your intensity until you are sprinting at
least the last 100 yards at your absolute maximum speed. You
should finish this last repeat with that totally 'blown out' feeling
you get from sprinting the last 100 yards of a race, which leaves
you gasping for breath and grabbing your knees for support."
Then watch your heart-rate monitor, or, better yet, have a friend
nearby who can watch the numbers for you. Then write down
your maximum.

"It's amazing how spacey a runner's mind gets doing a workout like this," Parker cautions. "So don't go through this whole
procedure and get back home only to realize sometime later in the
shower that you have no idea what your max number was."

If that is what it takes to get your heart to beat as fast as it
can, no wonder the heart-rate formula is inaccurate. How many

people, especially people who are not used to exercising, will ever push themselves to that extent? I wonder if it is even safe, especially for the middle-aged and elderly. Might some people be risking a heart attack trying to get that blown-out feeling?

The American College of Sports Medicine advises men over forty and women over fifty to have an exercise stress test before even trying vigorous exercise, and an attempt to find your maximum heart rate would certainly qualify as vigorous. Others are not so sure that such pre-exercise testing would make much of a difference. The American College of Cardiology and the American Heart Association say that the testing has not been shown to be useful.

The biggest risk is that atherosclerotic plaque may rupture and cause a heart attack, and that is of particular concern in the obese, smokers, people with high cholesterol levels, people with diabetes, and those who are the least physically active. Nonetheless, death during exercise is rare, and, for reasons that are uncertain, when it does occur, the victims usually are men.

Over the years, leading medical journals have published studies that attempted to determine how risky it is to exercise. Some asked how many heart-attack patients had been stricken while exercising, or soon afterwards. For example, Murray Mittleman, a professor of medicine at Harvard, did a study of 1,228 heart-attack patients, finding that 4.4 percent had engaged in strenuous exercise an hour before their attacks, but that the heart attack victims were mostly people who had been leading sedentary lives. In his 1993 paper in the *New England Journal of Medicine*, Mittleman establishes a rough risk estimate: if a fifty-year-old man who is sedentary but does not smoke and is not a diabetic engages in strenuous activity for an hour, his risk of having a heart attack in that hour will rise 100-fold over what it would be if he were not exercising. But even then, the paper notes, "his absolute risk in that hour would still be only 1 in 10,000."

Others investigated the risk of sudden death from a wildly abnormal heart rhythm brought on by vigorous exercise. One of the largest such studies, by JoAnn Manson, a professor of medicine at Harvard, examined 122 sudden deaths that occurred in a twelve-year period among 21,481 male doctors. In her findings, published in 2000 in the *New England Journal of Medicine*, she explained that the men were ages 40 to 84 when the study began and had not been diagnosed with heart disease. How many of those deaths occurred during or just after exercise, she asked, as compared to ones that occurred when the men were not exercising? She and her colleagues concluded that sudden death is about 17 times more likely with vigorous exercise; but even so, the risk is minuscule, with one death per 1.51 million vigorous exercise sessions. The risks were greatest in men who rarely or never exercised, and least in those who exercised five or more times a week.

Paul Thompson, a cardiologist and marathon runner who has reviewed all the published studies, concludes that the findings are consistent: the risk that someone will have a heart attack or die suddenly while exercising, or just afterwards, is small and is concentrated among sedentary men who have other risk factors, such as heart disease, obesity, and smoking.

So is it safe to just go for that blown-out feeling to find your maximum heart rate? Thompson and other cardiologists say that healthy men under age thirty-five and women under forty should be able to try it on their own, without seeing a doctor first. Older people who are sedentary or who have other conditions, such as being overweight or having diabetes or heart disease, should check with a doctor before trying it.

I'm over forty but I have no other risk factors, so I took a chance, going for that blown-out feeling, and found what I think is my maximum heart rate. Knowing it helps me exercise more vigorously. One night, I realized why it matters to me.

As I was leaving a Spinning class, I heard a young woman talking to the instructor, Arline Lohli. It was her first class, she said, and she was bored. In aerobics classes, she had to pay rapt attention to keep up with the steps and the dancelike patterns, but in Spinning you can spend five minutes just standing up straight and pedaling. Suddenly, I understood why Spinning is different for me and why I love it so much. It is because in Spinning I challenge myself by seeing how intensely I can push myself. And the higher I keep my heart rate, the more exhilarated I feel. It is that experience that draws me to exercise, and it is that feeling I start to crave when I go more than a few days between vigorous exercise sessions. It is a sensation that is hard to describe to someone who has not experienced it—it combines euphoria with a sort of clear-headedness and a feeling that I have somehow moved into another zone, like the feeling you might get when you are totally absorbed in your work, or in playing a musical instrument. It does not always come in a Spinning class, but I know that it can happen, and the way to get there is to strive for intense exertion. Being able to monitor my heart rate lets me work harder longer, and that is what helps get me to that state where I feel so good.

I recall Kirkendall's words: "Most people have no idea how hard they can work."

But working hard is not what many personal trainers and exercise-class instructors advocate for people who want to lose weight. They tell you to do something that sounds downright paradoxical: keep your heart rate low, they say, to burn fat. A moderate workout will help you lose more weight than an intense one. And therein lies another facet of the heart-rate obsession that permeates the exercise culture.

This odd-sounding notion that a slow heart rate helps you use your body's fat as fuel is enshrined on so many exercise machines, which prominently display "weight-loss zones" or "fat-burning zones" for your heart rate and often have programs that are supposed to keep you working at this moderate pace. More intense exercise is supposed to be reserved for "cardiovascular" training.

The idea is that if you want to get rid of fat, you should force your body to burn it. Muscles prefer to use sugar, in the form of glycogen, for energy, because it is so easy to metabolize. But they also can use fat. The fat-burning-zone hypothesis says that if you don't push yourself too hard, your muscles will burn fat and you will lose weight. Extreme exertion, however, will force your muscles to burn glycogen, leaving your body's fat intact.

When I check the Web site for Polar Electro, the heart-rate monitor company, I see allusions to the fat-burning zone in the "Research" section. There, in text written by the company, Polar states: "Reducing the amount of fat tissue in the body is an important target for those exercising for weight loss and weight management purposes." It adds: "the use of fat as an energy source is optimum (highest possible percentage) at the energy intensity of about 50 percent of maximal aerobic power, VO2max, and decreases thereafter." A chart lets you see not just where the optimum fat-burning zone is in terms of maximal aerobic power, but also in terms of heart rate. That turns out to be a heart rate that is about 60 percent of maximum.

Something about this hypothesis rings false. It seems to defy common sense, and many people find it hard to suspend their disbelief. Arline, the Gold's Gym Spinning instructor, has mentioned the fat-burning theory in all seriousness, but neither she nor the other thin and devoted exercisers seem to follow it. They are the ones who are working at the highest heart rates. And it is not as though these people all are naturally thin; many worry constantly about their weight. Yet, to hear them talk, it seems that the idea of low-intensity exercise never entered their minds.

Arline is angular and lean. A high school teacher with blond hair piled high on her head, she has a firm manner and she never smiles, but admonishes us: "If you can pedal faster than the beat of the music, you're cheating—turn up your resistance." And: "You. Should. Look. Like You're. Pushing." She warns us: "This next song, you're going to push your heart rates to the max." Her tough classes are one reason she is so popular.

One Saturday morning, we join Arline's regular Spinning crowd in her eight-thirty class. Halfway through, she announces that the next song will be our break, a chance to slow down for a few minutes and ease off on the resistance. "We don't want a break," shouts Laura, one of the gym's avid exercisers, from the front row of bikes, her usual spot in this, one of her usual classes. Most of us continue working just as hard, sacrificing the break. Forty minutes go by and the class is supposed to end. Arline asks if we want to keep going. We say yes. Do we want to sprint, she asks. Of course. So here it is, fifty minutes after the class began. The air conditioner is turned to its coldest setting, yet sweat is puddled on the floor around our bikes. Arline's sports bra, charcoal-gray stripes on a light-gray background, is dark with perspiration. Finally, the class draws to a close and we are doing the mandatory cleanup, wiping our bikes with paper towels sprayed with disinfectant, when Arline says, "Let's go weigh ourselves." A guy, walking out of the room, looks at her in puzzlement. "He doesn't get it," Arline says.

The rest of us, three women who are hard-core Spinning enthusiasts, know exactly what she means. Crazy at it sounds, here's the subtext: We did not eat before class—you can't eat much before a hard workout. And we saw the pools of sweat around our bikes. So we must be lighter.

It happens again on a Thursday in early December when Sandy shows up for class. He's a competitive bicyclist who sometimes uses Spinning to train on weekday nights, especially in the winter. I had thought that if there was one person who never thought about or worried about getting fat, it was Sandy. I was wrong.

I greet him as we arrange our bikes. Sandy is wearing one of his usual outfits, a skintight red bicycling jersey and skintight bicycling shorts. A computer science researcher, he was in Morocco for the past six days on business and he simply could not find a gym. He has had no exercise for a week, he says, and he is worrying about his weight. I look at him—if there is any fat on him, I certainly can't see it. His torso is narrow and his legs are densely muscled. He looks like he always does, like a man who was built for bicycling. All of his strength seems poured into his powerful legs, with their bulging quadriceps and rock-solid calves.

The class was challenging, led by an instructor, Claire Frazier, who pushed us relentlessly. Now it's over and we're wiping down our bikes. "I'm going to go weigh myself," Sandy says, smiling as he steps over the puddles of sweat on the floor.

Of course, if you believed in the fat-burning-zone idea, you would say that these thin people are deluding themselves. They would lose more fat if they did less.

And yet, as my husband likes to say, weight loss is a matter of simple physics. If you take in more calories than you use, you will gain weight. If you take in fewer calories than you use, you will lose weight. What difference should it make whether your body uses fat or carbohydrates as its primary energy source while you are exercising? The only thing that should matter is how many calories you burn. And the harder you work during the time you are exercising, the more energy you will use and so the more calories you will burn.

That certainly is true for diets, obesity researchers have found. Although diet fad after diet fad becomes popular—low fat, low carbohydrate, careful balancing of carbohydrates, protein, and fat—studies have repeatedly found that the only thing that matters is how many calories you take in, not where they come from. One of my favorites is a 1992 study in the *American Journal of Clinical Nutrition*, by Rudolph Leibel of Columbia University's College of Physicians and Surgeons and Jules Hirsch of Rockefeller University. Both were working at Rockefeller at the time, where their colleague, Pete Ahrens, was trying to see how cholesterol levels changed, if at all, when people ate different diets.

Leibel and Hirsch were interested in obesity and noticed that a study by Ahrens provided them with data to ask how the composition of a diet might affect weight gain. Ahrens had put over-weight people in a metabolic-study ward of a hospital and had given them meals that were carefully designed to be mostly car-bohydrate or mostly fat. He knew exactly what the subjects were eating, he knew exactly how many calories they were burning each day, and he had carefully titrated the amount of food each person got in order to keep each person's weight constant. He was looking at their cholesterol levels and finding that while some responded to a high-fat diet with rising cholesterol levels, others did not. Leibel and Hirsch noticed something else: it took the same number of calories of fat as it took of carbohydrates to maintain each person's weight. The source of the calories made no difference—all that mattered was the number of calories.

So if the simple physics argument says that the source of your body's fuel makes no difference in controlling your weight, that all that matters is how much fuel you put into your body, why wouldn't it also explain the other side of the equation? Why should it matter *how* you burn calories, whether by walking or running?

It turns out that the myth of low-intensity-exercise fat burning is a misunderstanding of a basic relationship, best seen on a graph. One line shows muscles' use of fat as an energy source as a function of exercise intensity, and another line depicts muscles' use of carbohydrates as a function of exercise intensity. The crossover point, where equal amounts of fat and carbohydrate are being burned, comes at about 60 percent of your maximum effort, or a heart rate that is about 70 percent of maximum. After that, the amount of carbohydrate burned exceeds the amount of fat, and this imbalance increases as exercise intensity increases. If you get to your maximum heart rate, less than ten percent of the calories you burn will come from fat.

That led to the argument that as long as you keep your heart rate low enough, you will burn more fat than carbohydrates and you will lose more weight. The problem is that the argument is neglecting a crucial component: the number of calories burned.

The harder you work, the more energy you expend, and the more calories you will need.

Jack Wilmore of Texas A&M and Dave Costill of Ball State provide the example of a twenty-five-year-old woman. One day, she exercises for half an hour at a low intensity (she walks) and burns half her 220 calories as fat. The next day, she exercises for half an hour at a higher intensity (moderately paced running) and burns just a third of her 332 calories as fat.

"The total calories from fat do not differ between the low and high intensity workouts," write Wilmore and Costill. "In both cases, she burns about 110 calories of fat during 30 minutes. Most important, however, for the higher-intensity workout, she expends about 50 percent more total calories for the same time period!"

I do a little test on the elliptical trainer, which displays the rate you are burning calories as you exercise. It takes into account your weight (a larger person, of course, burns more than a smaller person), the amount of resistance on the pedals, and the speed you are moving. When I was exercising at the low end of the "weight-loss" range, the machine said I was burning 6.5 calories a minute. At the high end of that range, I burned 10 calories a minute. When I worked a little harder and got into the "cardiovascular" range, the calories per minute ranged from 10 at the low end to 14 at the top of that range. That means that I would burn more than twice as many calories if I kept my heart rate at the top of the cardiovascular range than I would if I stayed at the bottom of the weight-loss range.

It seems so obvious that the fat-burning zone idea is wrong that I wonder where it came from. No one seems to provide any references to research papers advocating it. Is it an urban legend of the fitness industry, I ask Costill. As one of the grand old men of the exercise physiology world, he might at least remember when and how the notion got started. He confirms my suspicions, remarking, "I'm not sure that the fat-burning concept at low exercise intensities can be blamed on any one person."

I check with Wilmore, who also has seen the exercise movement burgeon. He believes it began in the late 1970s or early eighties with the aerobic dance movement. From there, he recalls, it spread rapidly, permeating the exercise culture. Before long, the idea took on the air of received wisdom among exercisers and those who provide exercise advice.

"Like many fads in the exercise-dieting game, things look a lot better in theory than in practice," Wilmore says.

five

TRAINING LORE

Heart-rate monitors in hand, Bill and I get our schedule for the Mount Everest ride—a stapled handful of photocopied pages that are a mixture of fear-inducing instructions and detailed training advice. I look first at the part called "The Day of the Event." We are told to "bring sandals to walk around in since the floor will be slippery" and to bring "plastic bags for wet clothes."

Yet for a ride that could be so grueling that by the time it is over the entire floor might be slick with sweat, the training does not look very hard. It is supposed to get us ready to ride for four hours on a Saturday afternoon in April 2001. But in the eleven weeks leading up to the ride, all we have to do is lift weights two times a week, take three Spinning classes during the week, and do one long Spinning ride each weekend. The weekend rides are to last from one to three hours, getting longer and longer as we get closer to the actual Mount Everest ride. I had thought we would be asked to do more—train with rides that were longer than the usual forty to forty-five minutes during the week, or train with some very fast rides or some rides with very high resistance on our pedals to teach us to endure as we climbed long hills. Yet, when I look at the instructions it seems that training for Mount Everest will not be much different than what we are doing already, with our week-night habit of Spinning classes and our regular weight-lifting sessions.

Maybe, I think, training is just one of those exercise myths. Maybe training only matters at the very top end of the scale, for elite athletes who have to shave seconds off an already fast time to compete. Maybe it makes no difference for people like Bill and me; and maybe we could just go out and ride for four hours any time we choose.

I mention my idea to Kathryn Schwartz, one of the Spinning instructors who was planning the Mount Everest ride.

"You could ride for four hours right now," Kathryn says. "You could get through it. But you would not feel very good afterward." She is a serious distance bicyclist, going out on the roads with a cycling club that thinks little of riding 100 miles in a day and that almost never cancels a ride no matter how bad the weather. She even rode 200 miles once, on a day that featured one thunderstorm after another—seven storms in all. But I don't know whether to believe her about training. Her pale blond hair is cut short for easy care—by some odd quirk, virtually every woman who teaches Spinning at our gym is blond—but she is not a hard-driving, lanky woman like her fellow instructor Arline. Kathryn has a gentleness about her, a soft voice and a mild manner. And, unlike Arline, she does not have the look of a maximum-heart-rate fanatic. Her body is rounded, although firm, and she favors long black tights that seem as if they would be uncomfortably hot in a tough class. Yet Kathryn does do those long outdoor rides, she does train. And I have never done anything like Mount Everest.

The only time I trained for anything was fifteen years earlier, when two colleagues of mine at *Science* magazine told me how much fun it was to run in the annual ten-mile Cherry Blossom Race in Washington, D.C. They were faster runners than I, so even though they had invited me, I knew I would be on my own.

I trained alone, following the instructions I found in a book at the library, *The Beauty of Running*, by Gayle Barron and Kim Chapin (published in 1980, it is now out of print). I liked the picture of the woman runner on the cover, athletic and glowing with health. I would go out for long runs along a bike path that hugged the edge of MacArthur Boulevard, a road that went from the end of my block in Washington out to the suburbs. The Potomac River was on my left as I ran toward Maryland, and adjacent to it was the flat brown water of the Chesapeake and Ohio Canal. The trees were starting to bud, the air was soft, and it was easy to daydream as I ran. I always followed the same path and I did just what the book said, steadily increasing my distance, not worrying about speed, until finally, the week before the race, I went for ten miles.

But it took me only eighty minutes to run the Cherry Blossom Race. That is very different from an event like Mount Everest that lasts for four hours. I had no idea whether training that included trying to go fast, at least some days of the week, would have made me run faster. And I had no idea whether I could have run that race without training, just by continuing my usual runs that were never longer than five or six miles.

Almost as soon as Bill and I sign up for Mount Everest, I have a chance to test my idea that I am already trained for it. Gold's Gym announces that it is sponsoring a three-hour Spinning ride to raise money for charity. Bill and I have not trained for the charity ride, of course, but neither has anyone else—it is supposed to be fun, not a testimony to your assiduous preparation. Yet it might serve as a comparison for what a long ride feels like before and after training.

We arrive on a Saturday morning for the three-hour ride, wearing our skintight black bicycling shorts with special padded crotches, and take our seats in a circle of twenty bikes. The instructors are the trio of blondes—Arline Lohli, Anna Hess, and Kathryn Schwartz. The bikes are filled with familiar people. Sandy, the competitive cyclist, is the most impressive. He comes lugging a gym bag crammed with food and sports drinks to sustain him and with extra towels and two extra jerseys so he can strip off his sweaty shirt every hour and replace it with a fresh one.

I greet Sam Bruno, a densely muscled man with short silver hair and a fleshy face. He favors sleeveless white T-shirts for his Gold's Gym workouts, and a sand-colored baseball cap. On the top of his left arm, at the level of his deltoid muscle, is a tattoo of a black cat against an orange moon. He has another tattoo on his back, at waist level, of a turtle. Sam is, as always, friendly and full of advice. He tells me that he has done a three-hour ride. It's easy, he says. Just pace yourself, don't push too hard—advice I have no intention of following, of course. Exercise, to me, means pushing.

After the first hour, Bill and I are stunned by our physiological response. It is becoming progressively harder to keep our heart rates up and to force our legs to push the pedals. By the beginning of the third hour, my heart rate is ten beats per minute below where it was after the warm-up at the start of the class—it has plummeted below what I think of as my target zone—and I am struggling just to keep going.

I ask Steve Nissen, the cardiologist at the Cleveland Clinic, what might have happened to me. "Maybe your heart got tired," he said. My heart? I could not believe it. I had thought that hearts never get tired, and somehow Nissen's suggestion is much scarier than the idea that my muscles gave out or I somehow lost my motivation. How can a heart get tired?

I later discover that Sam and his wife, Kathy Bruno, also find these long rides almost unendurable. I come across Sam and Kathy beside the cable-pulley machine at the gym one evening. Kathy is a ponytailed, gum-chewing Spinning instructor with a turtle tattoo to match her husband's and an infectious grin. I never imagined she would have trouble with a three-hour ride. But she tells me that when she first tried one, she was as tired as I was. She went home and slept for an hour. Then, she says "When I got up, I was so hungry I just ate all day." Sam says that after the first hour of his first three-hour ride, he was so exhausted that he wanted to leave. He stayed on only because he did not want to embarrass himself by being the only one to quit.

Bill and I had the same sort of experience. We dragged ourselves off of our bikes when the ride finally ended and drove
home. I stretched out on our soft brown sofa to read the newspaper, my head propped up by two throw pillows. I did not want to
admit it, but all I really wanted to do was sleep. Bill was in pain—
his hip flexor muscles started aching right after the ride and did
not stop hurting for two days. If this was what a three-hour fun
ride is like, how are we ever going to get through Mount Everest?
Or will we feel differently after we train?

Skeptic that I am, the first thing I notice about training is that
coaches do not always agree on how to do it. I look over some
training programs for marathons—I have toyed with the idea of
running one, so I have a little collection of advice on how to
train—and I see that each marathon expert has a different plan.

The Boston Athletic Association has a sixteen-week program
that suggests learning to go fast by running in several long races
of ten to twenty miles and setting aside a day each week for interval training—fast running for distances of half a mile to two
miles, interspersed with periods where you run more slowly. To
gain endurance, you are supposed to run each day and include
"medium-long runs" of ten to fourteen miles every other week.
You are supposed to let your body recover before the marathon
by tapering—easing off on training—for the last three weeks.

Hal Higdon, who trains marathon runners in Chicago, has an
eighteen-week program based on one long run each week, gradually building up to twenty miles in length. The long run is followed by a day of cross-training—doing some other sport like
walking, bicycling, or swimming to recover. You get one or two
rest days each week; the other days you run, but shorter distances
than the long run. He favors walking breaks and says that his
group, which trains by running along Lake Michigan in Chicago,
stops and walks every mile or so, striding or, perhaps, ambling up
to the water fountains that are spaced at about one-mile intervals.

But he does not tell runners to enter other races during their marathon training—they can learn to run faster by actually running faster once a week, he says.

The New York City Road Runners Club gives advice on how to train for the New York Marathon. Like the others, they advocate one long run every week and, like the Boston group, suggest entering races, urging runners to race at least once a month, though no more than twice in a month. Unlike the others, the New York group tells runners they can use "running equivalents" (another term for cross-training) for up to 25 percent of their training, substituting a sport that does not pound their legs and feet. The New York coaches suggest riding a bike or swimming for this alternate exercise, but urge runners to keep their heart rates as high as they would be if they were running and to do these alternate exercises for the same length of time that they would run.

I was looking for a formula, a recipe for success that would turn an untrained person into a marathoner. And I was finding a general pattern—long runs once a week, a rest day every week— discernible in the training programs that each individual coach seems to have invented. Then again, when I hear stories that athletes tell of how they trained, there are usually lots of anecdotes but little science.

There are the competitive walkers, starting, of course, with one of the original champions, the celebrated pedestrian Captain Alardice Barclay. In the early 1800s, Barclay set a record, completing a 1,000-mile walk in 1,000 hours. His eccentric training plan consisted of days filled with long walks and short sprints, and meals of rare beef or mutton with stale bread and old beer.

Two hundred years later, another walker, Brian Robertson, invented his own training program. On October 27, 2001, he accomplished walking's triple crown: Robertson became the first person to hike the Appalachian Trail, the Pacific Crest Trail, and the Continental Divide Trail in a single year, a distance of 7,371 miles, which he completed in just ten months. A forty-year-old computer scientist and competitive hiker, Robertson trained for two years before attempting his long hike, running fifty miles a week until the last three months before the walk began, when he ran ninety miles a week. He calculated what he would eat, planning on 6,000 calories a day. "I eat food," he said, "I don't taste it." During his hike, he ate every two hours, devouring whole chickens and whole cheesecakes in the evening, wolfing down two quarts of ice cream at lunch time, eating three Snickers bars a day for a total of 900 bars during his 300-day solitary journey.

For bicycling, I find some very odd training advice in the April 1946 issue of *Bicycling* magazine. Athletes were advised to "walk rapidly for about half a mile but carrying the bicycle with your arm cocked so that the bicycle's cross bow is just off your shoulders. This tends to throw your shoulders back and stretches your chest and lungs, developing your grip, wrists, and arms. Change arms in carrying at will, but at no time during your set distance for this exercise let the bike touch the ground or your shoulder." The article suggests making the exercise more challenging by setting up competitions, "seeing who can carry their bicycle the farthest, or race to a given point under the above rules."

Then there are the runners. Clarence DeMar, the champion marathon runner at the beginning of the twentieth century, bought a small book by the Spaulding Company on distance runs "and studied it carefully." Running to and from work to train, he put in seven to fourteen miles a day. But he was not averse to experimenting. He received a letter from a Dr. Kellogg of Battle Creek, Michigan (not, by the way, the Kellogg of cornflakes fame), who wanted him to try a special training diet that forbade meat. DeMar agreed, although he found it a bit awkward at times to follow the program.

"When I went away from home or anyone visited us, it was embarrassing to have to explain about my eating habits," he said, adding that "I felt my running would be more justified if I contributed something to the noble experiment of science!"

On the day of the Boston Marathon, DeMar ate exactly as
Kellogg had instructed him: a dozen oranges, a quarter-pound of
pine nuts, and a pound of caramels. "I found that it took nearly
the whole morning to eat all this stuff," he wrote. "After this
marathon of eating, I didn't feel especially full of pep." Nonetheless, he won the race. Yet he was not altogether convinced of the
value of Dr. Kellogg's training diet: "At heart, I couldn't get away
from the thought that I probably would have won anyhow and
that if the experiment had any scientific value it was simply to
show that a person could have plenty of endurance without meat
for some months."

One of the greatest runners ever, Czechoslovakian Emil Zapotek, devised some of the most extreme ways to train himself.
He ran through knee-deep snow in army boots. He dashed down
the street, from telephone pole to telephone pole, holding his
breath. He ran with his wife, Dana, on his shoulders. He ran in
place for hours, reading a book or listening to the radio. He put
dirty clothes in his bathtub and ran on them.

Some of the stories of Zapotek's training are surely apoc-
ryphal; still, other runners, believing them, tried in vain to dupli-
cate them. It was said that he ran sixty quarter-mile sprints in a
row, doing each in sixty seconds, a feat beyond known human
ability. Yet his competitors, believing Zapotek succeeded, tried to
do it themselves. After all, other runners reasoned, something in
Zapotek's training must have made him great. His triumphs were
legendary. In 1952, he ran in the Helsinki Olympics and won the
5,000-meter race, the 10,000-meter race, and the marathon, each
time setting an Olympic record. He had never run a marathon before, yet finished in two hours, twenty-three minutes, and four
seconds, two and a half minutes ahead of the second-place fin-
isher. When that runner entered the Olympic stadium, he was
confronted with the sight of Zapotek munching an apple and
chatting with his wife.

Another legendary runner, champion distance runner Ted
Corbitt, who raced in marathons and ultramarathons and even

twenty-four-hour races, was inspired by Zapotek. He invented his own training programs and experimented to see what worked best. But unlike Zapotek, who often frolicked with his wife when he trained, Corbitt liked to be alone.

Dave Costill, the veteran exercise physiologist at Ball State, studied Corbitt in 1967, when Corbitt was forty-six, giving him treadmill tests to learn how fast his heart beat and how much oxygen he used while running at different speeds, even giving him psychological tests in an attempt to understand what made him so great. Corbitt, he tells me, had what he believes is a typical personality for a distance runner. The man was "the ultimate introvert. You could sit in a room with him for four hours and he would never say a word. You might be uncomfortable, but he wouldn't." His training was grueling, consisting of endless hours of solitary running.

Corbitt was running 100 miles a week to train for his first marathon, in 1951, when he decided that his training had to include at least one 30-mile run if he was to race for 26 miles. The first few times he tried to go for 30 miles, he gave up at 20 or 22 miles, but finally, one winter day, he had a revelation.

"It was a snowy February day and I set out to try for thirty again. I started to get thirsty and stuck out my tongue to catch some snowflakes. I did this all through the run and that day broke through to thirty miles. It was those snowflakes, the water that did it. I never drank water before on my runs and now realized that I was terribly dehydrated. From that day on I always made sure I was properly hydrated."

He also tried unusual foods. In 1973, when he was fifty-four, he was invited to participate in a twenty-four-hour race in England. His trainer, he said, "developed a concoction consisting of two hard-boiled eggs mashed in a cup of orange juice, which could be swallowed easily. Intermittent treats of chocolate bars, orange and pineapple slices, blackberry juice, and a can of sardines rounded out the gourmet menu." He downed it as he raced. And afterward, his trainer "had a special technique for alleviating stiffness, by stroking my legs with a hard hairbrush to release neural energy. It worked."

But mostly Corbitt ran, unimaginable distances, day after day. He trained for a 50-mile race by running the 31 miles around Manhattan twice a day. Training for other races, he ran to and from his work as a physical therapist.

"I incorporated my training into my day, running twelve miles one way to work from my home in upper Manhattan to the Institute for the Crippled and Disabled. Sometimes I'd lengthen the route to twenty miles one way, depending on my schedule," Corbitt said. A taciturn man, he revealed little in interviews about why he did it. In a 1970 interview with Dave Costill and Edward L. Fox, another Ball State exercise physiologist, he remarked: "When I first started running distance races, I was motivated by the enjoyment of competition and a natural sensation of playing. Today, I run because my day just isn't complete unless I have run twenty to thirty miles. I am also driven by a fear that if I ever stop running for any period of time, I may never be able to get started again."

But at least Corbitt's decision to undergo these grueling runs was his own. Some college athletes had little choice, their coaches having invented training programs that they imposed upon anyone who wanted to compete for their school.

In 1977, Ron Richardson, the newly hired men's track coach at the University of Wyoming, was determined to make the team a national powerhouse. To force his runners to run faster, he would tie a rope to a belt around the runner's waist and hold the other end of the rope himself as he drove his Volkswagon Beetle up and down mountain roads. When his cross-country team lost one of its meets, he drove the young men seventeen miles out of town and made them run home. He brought in runners from Kenya who were older than the rest of the team and already champions, making them members of the team and throwing the younger men into daily exhausting and disheartening competitions with these seasoned athletes. In the end, Richardson had success: his cross-country team placed third in the nation that year. But whether it was his training program or the infusion of Kenyans is open to question.

What is possibly the ultimate in training stories is the saga of how Bernd Heinrich, a biology professor at the University of Vermont, made up a program that resulted in his setting a world record for a race of 100 kilometers (62.137 miles) on an asphalt pavement in Chicago on October 4, 1981. His time was a blistering 6 hours, 38 minutes, and 21 seconds.

Heinrich was no novice. He had been running since he was ten, and had run marathons and even a 50-kilometer race. But in 1980 he had turned forty and was beginning to worry that his best years were behind him, noting that Costill had said that distance runners peak between the ages of twenty-seven and thirty-two. The next fall, when he would turn forty-one, the U.S. National Championship 100-kilometer race would be held. "Go for it now or you'll regret it forever, my mind said back then," he recalled.

Heinrich knew that he had to find a way to train that would change his body's physiology, to make it capable of the feat. "I had to remodel myself with the constraints of my 'normal physiology' to be able to do what would not otherwise be possible." He was living in a tarpaper shack in the Maine woods during the spring and summer before the race. He knew of no training manuals for a 100-kilometer race. But he realized what the challenges would be. He asked himself how he would get enough fuel to his muscles since, he notes, "to run 62.2 miles would be to enter the body's carbohydrate-fuel-depletion zone twice over." He wanted to conserve energy while he ran—even to use as little energy as possible in breathing. As a biologist, he started asking himself: What are the speed and endurance secrets of antelopes, of honeybees, of camels? Could he adapt them to his own training?

Heinrich began training himself in early May of 1981, running 15 to 17 miles several days in a row. To his surprise, he discovered he was getting weaker. "That was frightening. Then I figured

it out. I noticed that along with my fatigue came hunger, sometimes intense hunger. There were several times that I got so weak
and hungry that I knocked at a stranger's door, begging for a slice
of dry bread." Yet eventually he would run up to 20 miles a day,
day after day, without eating much more than he did before his
training began and without feeling weak from hunger. The only
explanation, he figured, was that he had trained his body to be
more efficient, in both how it moved and how it used calories.

He also worried about endurance and decided that not only
would he undertake long runs at the beginning and end of the day
but also shorter runs at noon and sometimes even a short run before or after his long run. Beyond that, "I wanted to make my
body think it had to run all the time. I never walked. Even if I
needed to go only fifty yards to the library or to my car, I jogged.
My body must not be allowed to think it would ever walk again."

Now there was the problem of what to eat during the run.
Heinrich considered drinking honey, noting that a honeybee car-
ries honey equal to its body weight in its crop and uses it to fuel
flights that can last as long as three hours. But when he had tried
drinking a quart of honey before a run, it made him ill. He also
tried drinking olive oil, with a similarly disastrous result. He tried
beer—once again he got sick while he was running. He tried
candy bars and sandwiches but found he could not down them
while he ran because his mouth was too dry. Finally, he fixed on
cranberry juice, a liquid that is mostly sugar and water, like di-
luted honey.

Looking still to animals, birds, and insects for clues, Heinrich
decided not to stretch or lift weights. "I had never seen or heard
of an antelope who was flexible and did stretching or who lifted
weights for extra strength."

Just before the race, Heinrich decided to attempt to deplete his
muscles and liver of glycogen, their carbohydrate fuel, and then,
just before the race, stuff them full again by eating nothing but
carbohydrates. He thought he'd trust in the theory that such a
program would enable him to start the race with more glycogen

in his liver and muscles than they would ordinarily carry. After eating almost nothing but fats—butter, peanut butter, cheese, and fatty meat—for days, he felt nauseated; but that, he decided, was the only way to purge his body of glycogen. Two days before the race, he switched to eating nothing but carbs—bread, pasta, cookies, cereal. Then he and his wife flew to Chicago for the race, carrying pasta in a jar and yeast rolls for the pre-race meals. During the race he drank cranberry juice.

He won. Still, in retrospect he feels he made "foolish mistakes. I had not, for example, taken the findings from birds into account; I should have rested up more, carbo-depleted less, and taken a little protein on the run."

In the end, none of this makes much sense, and the training stories of athletes, from Captain Barclay down through Heinrich, only show me that people seem to be capable of extreme illogic in a quest for extreme fitness.

It turns out that while champion athletes are, of course, at the far end of what is humanly possible, most people are capable of changing their body's ability to perform by constantly demanding more and more of themselves.

The science involves understanding what happens to the body when you train—how your muscles change, why you get faster and stronger. It does not involve an actual recipe that results in the maximum training effect. "Training, to my knowledge, is not scientifically tested," Dave Costill tells me. "It's just trial and error." As a result, one can find some pretty strange programs. As Fritz Hagerman, an exercise physiologist at Ohio University put it: "There are a lot of myths. And the higher the stakes, the greater the myths." Training, he says, "is not a major science."

Training regimens have long been invented by coaches and athletes, and when they seemed to work, others would copy them. The one method that actually seems to be effective, that physically changes people's bodies, making them move faster and enabling them to exercise for longer and longer periods without tiring, was discovered in the 1930s by German physiologist Hans Rendell and a coach who worked with him, Woldemar Gerschler.

At the time, athletes were training by what was called "over-distance"—going farther than they would in their event. A runner who was going to run five miles might train by running ten. Rendell and Gerschler decided to try something different, a method they called "interval training." Working with runners, they asked athletes to repeatedly sprint, then recover by slowing down. According to their thinking, the most important training occurred in these recovery periods, the intervals. To include intervals in training, they proposed, would make the heart stronger and better able to deliver oxygen-rich blood to the muscles. Rendell and Gerschler insisted that a runner's heart rate must drop to 120 beats a minute during the intervals. They claimed, furthermore, that if the athlete's heart rate did not get this low within 90 seconds, the workout was too hard.

The plan was to map out a year-long schedule, starting with ten months in which the runners were preparing for the two-month racing season. The athletes would start with what is now called base-building, developing a foundation of endurance by running long distances each day. Then they would build speed with interval training, doing sprints between short recovery periods. As they spent more time on interval training, the runners cut back on endurance training.

To demonstrate the value of their method, Rendell and Gerschler selected a young runner, Rudolph Harbig. They trained him and the results were spectacular. In 1939, he ran an 800-meter race in 1 minute 46.6 seconds, lopping 1.6 seconds off the previous world record. A few weeks later, Harbig broke the world record for the 400-meter run, with a time of 46 seconds. Harbig's 800-meter record lasted for sixteen years, falling only when another Gerschler-trained runner, Roger Moens, covered the same distance in 1 minute 45.7 seconds.

Harbig, of course, was naturally gifted, as Fritz Hagerman

points out. "They picked the right person," he says of Rendell and Gerschler. "He was magnificent."

Today, runners have gotten so good that Harbig's incredible 800-meter time wouldn't even guarantee him a win at the National College Athletic Association championships. The world record now is 1 minute 41 seconds. And interval training is inscribed in textbooks.

But the revolutionary interval-training method was nearly lost during World War II. It is demanding, and easy to neglect if coaches feel they are doing fine with their old ways. The overdistance approach remained the method of choice.

"We were so traditional—most of the training was whatever was good for the coaches," Hagerman explained. For runners, the training was simple. "You would run a couple of hours to train."

Interval training reemerged—or maybe it was rediscovered independently—in the 1950s when a medical student at Oxford University, Roger Gilbert Bannister, did what was long thought to be physiologically impossible: he ran a mile in under four minutes. His time, on May 6, 1954, was 3 minutes 59.4 seconds.

As Bannister drew close to the finish line, he knew the stakes: "The arms of the world were waiting to receive me if only I reached the tape without slackening my speed. If I faltered, there would be no arms to hold me and the world would be a cold, forbidding place because I was so close."

His coach was Franz Stampfl, a former skier from Vienna who had fled Austria just after the Berlin Olympics in 1936. Before his death in 1995, in an interview on Australian radio, he claimed credit for inventing interval training: "I developed a form of running which is called 'interval training,' which took me more than twenty years or more to put into practice the first time, or successfully, with Roger Bannister." The reason it worked, he explained, was that it was "a stress adaptation."

Gradually, more and more coaches began using the method. Hagerman was converted in the 1960s. He had just taken a Ph.D.

in exercise physiology at Ohio State and his family and he wanted an adventure. "There was an opportunity to go to New Zealand and teach at the medical school." There, in Auckland, Hagerman found himself intrigued by the success of a track coach, Arthur Lydiard, who coached several runners who had seemed talented, though hardly extraordinary. After training with Lydiard, however, they went on to set world records, in races ranging from 800 meters to marathons.

"These people were survivors of a very, very difficult training process," Hagerman observed. "This was before people began doing really hard workouts. Even his middle-distance runners ran well over 100 miles a week. And he introduced interval training to his runners." Although there was a general belief by then that the method worked, it seemed so grueling that "people were reluctant to use it."

Around this time, members of a local rowing club paid Hagerman a visit. They wanted to know if he would work with them and train them the way Lydiard trained his runners. "I said, 'I don't know anything about rowing.'" But he set out to watch the young men. "I was immediately impressed by just the power outputs they were able to generate and the training they performed," he says. He began working with the rowers, introducing them to endurance training and interval training, and went on to make rowing the focus of his research career. He wanted to find out what made rowers improve and why some were so much better than others. As part of his work, he documented over and over again that rowers who used interval training became stronger and faster. Interval training was so effective, in fact, that the real danger was that athletes would overshoot, reaching their peak ability before their race.

"You've got to be very careful about using it," Hagerman says.

He was not alone in trying the interval training method. At about the same time Hagerman was working with rowers, Costill began trying the method with cross-country runners. He knew little about running; he had been a swimmer in college in the 1950s, and that was the only sport he understood well. But his own training had been fairly relaxed. The team would practice by simply emphasizing different parts of their stroke for distances of 400 meters (about a quarter-mile). "You'd swim a 400, kick a 400, pull a 400. That was about it," Costill recalled. "We did some speed work but not much. We'd take two hours and maybe do a mile."

Costill ended up coaching cross country from 1964 through 1966, while finishing his Ph.D. in exercise physiology. He had landed a teaching job at the State University of New York at Cortland, where the training philosophy was just to run for long distances.

"It didn't matter how fast they ran," Costill says. "They'd just train 'L.S.D.'—long slow distance." The result, he said, was predictable. "Your endurance would be good, but you just wouldn't have any speed."

He noticed that some swimming coaches were starting to use interval training, and some track coaches were adopting it to train sprinters. Costill decided to try interval training with his cross-country runners, whose races were five miles long. It worked. In the two seasons that Costill coached them, the Cortland team was suddenly a powerhouse, winning seven out of ten meets in 1964 and every race in 1965. Cortland's yearbook, in recognition of the team's spectacular record in 1964, notes admiringly that Costill "sent his runners through one of the hardest training periods possible."

Now it is difficult to find training schedules that do not include some version of endurance and speed work. Heinrich achieved his amazing speed in the 100-kilometer race with just endurance training. But for most athletes, as well as for those who just want to do better in a race or an event like Mount Everest, the method has definitely taken hold. Donald Kirkendall, an exercise physiologist at the University of North Carolina, explains it simply: "If you want to push performance you've got to push the intensity." Yet there is a point of diminishing returns, when more exercise actually makes your performance worse.

Costill saw that for himself in the 1980s, when he looked at the performance of the Ball State swimming team and wondered if they were training too much. Like most teams then and now, they were working out twice a day.

It was January, halfway through the season, when the coach took Costill aside and said, "These guys have been training twice a day for three months or more. How much better will they get?" Costill replied that it was unlikely that they would get much better, at which point the coach said to him, "Then why are we doing it?"

Costill proposed an experiment. The next season, divide the team in half. One group would continue to train twice a day; the others would train just once a day. The swimmers who trained half as much improved dramatically, but the others got no better. The entire team switched to once-a-day training and began winning all their meets.

The reason that training works is the same reason that too much training can actually make performance worse, Costill explains. Training is a way of stressing the body. By forcing yourself to work longer or harder than you used to, you slightly injure your bodily systems. They respond by repairing the injuries, and they go one step farther, making the body just a bit stronger than it was before.

"The purpose of training is to tear the system down so that when you rest you'll be stronger than when you started," Costill says. "You allow the muscles to regenerate and regrow. Every cell when it is stressed will try to reinforce itself, so that if you stress it again it will grow stronger. But when you train day after day you have an accumulation of fatigue or cellular breakdown." The repair mechanisms have little chance to complete their work. But old habits die hard.

"The coaches are afraid to experiment. If for the last twenty years you've been training your swimmers four hours a day and

now someone comes along and says you can get the same results—or better results—with two hours a day, you have to admit
you've been wrong for twenty years. Coaches don't want to hear
that. Their egos get in the way. They would argue against it. But
they had much better swimmers, and we beat them."

There is no formula to predict when training becomes over-
training, Costill emphasizes. Some people can thrive on training
schedules that would destroy others. That is the danger of looking at legendary athletes like Ted Corbitt, with his training runs
around Manhattan—workouts that would break an ordinary
human. A good coach "knows when certain kids are breaking
down," Costill says. "You've got the best measure in the world,
the stopwatch. When kids perform poorly, most coaches will tell
them to work more. But it's not because they aren't training hard
enough. It's because they are training too hard."

While exercise physiologists and coaches have discovered regimens that work, some scientists are still asking why—what exactly happens to the body when a person trains? Why are some
people natural sprinters and others natural distance athletes? And
why do some people respond differently to training than others?

Exercise physiologists, comparing people before and after
training, learned that training makes the cardiovascular system
get better at delivering blood to muscles during exercise and it
makes the heart recover more quickly, making the pulse plummet
when effort decreases. The muscles also change, developing more
blood vessels so they can receive more blood. Within the muscles,
mitochondria, which are microscopic energy factories, multiply,
enabling the muscles to work harder. They store more glycogen,
their sugary energy source, enabling them to work longer without
tiring. And the muscles become more efficient in burning fat, another source of energy for them.

Some researchers began to focus on the muscles, asking
whether the key to efficient training might be to most effectively

alter muscle physiology. They knew the basics: muscles are composed of long, parallel strings of cells, the muscle fibers. Running along the length of each fiber are several hundred to several thousand myofibrils, which are long structures containing proteins that make a muscle contract. These proteins, actin and myosin, are arranged in long strings and rachet along each other. Duke University biologist Steven Vogel, author of *Prime Mover: A Natural History of Muscle*, likens the general mechanism to hauling something toward you "by pulling, arm over arm, on a long rope."

They also knew that muscles are specialized: some contract quickly, although they also run out of fuel quickly. Those are valuable for power and speed. Others contract more slowly but have a more plentiful energy supply, allowing them to keep going for long periods. Those are valuable for endurance. There also is a third type, intermediate between the two extremes. But why, some asked, even have different muscle types? And are these muscle types immutable, or can you change a muscle meant for endurance to one meant for speed? In other words, can you turn, say, a marathon runner into a sprinter?

Lawrence C. Rome, a biologist at the University of Pennsylvania, got interested in muscle types when he was a graduate student in the 1970s. "There is a feeling in evolutionary physiology that the properties of muscle fibers are very well matched to the tasks they have to perform." A muscle that must keep going for long periods of time, for example, will be very different from one called on only occasionally for short, intense bursts of effort, like sprinting. But Rome quickly learned that he could not get answers to questions about muscle types by studying humans, or even mammals. The problem, Rome explains, is that every muscle in a mammal is a combination of fiber types.

"If you wanted to figure out which ones were actually being used in slow running as compared to fast running, you could stick an electrode into the muscle during running and record the activity. But you could see an obvious problem—there are three mus-

cle fiber types surrounding the electrode and you have no way
of knowing which is causing the electrical activity," Rome says.
"You can't determine what muscle types power an activity because they're all interspersed."

The solution, he decided, was to study fish and frogs. "If you
go to a seafood store and look at swordfish, you see big patches
of white muscle and often see some small patches of dark meat.
These are the two major fiber types—the white is fast-twitch and
the red is slow-twitch." And, like humans and other animals, fish
often have an intermediate muscle fiber type, which is pinkish,
Rome adds. But the difference between fish and mammals, or
other animals, is that in fish, the fiber types are separated. The
white part of a fish is all fast-twitch and the red is all slow. Its red
color is due to the fact that it has a rich blood supply to provide
oxygen, whereas white muscle, which is anaerobic and uses
stored glycogen for energy, requires less blood.

The basic design of each muscle type is a compromise. In red
muscle, the cells are packed with mitochondria, their tiny self-
contained energy factories. But with as much as a third of the
space taken up by mitochondria, there is less room for the myofibrils, the chains of actin and myosin, proteins that slide up and
down, causing muscle to contract. White muscles do not have
many mitochondria, giving them more room for fibers, but the
trade-off is that they have a limited energy supply, and when it is
used up the muscle has to rest. In muscle, Rome says, "there is a
war for space."

The muscle fiber distribution in fish seems odd, though. If a
fish is going to swim all day, why does it have so much white
(fast-twitch) muscle and so little red? Rome explains that fish, living in water, are naturally buoyant and so they can carry a lot of
white muscle with little effort. It exists as a kind of reserve, used
only when needed for quick bursts of energy—to escape from
predators, for example.

"Fish use their red muscle 99.99 percent of the time," Rome
says. "They use their white muscle only once a day or once a

week." But when they use it, they need a lot of it. To accelerate quickly against the drag of water, they have to increase their power output fifty- or even a hundred-fold. "Each gram of white muscle generates twice as much power as a gram of red muscle," Rome says. "To increase the power fifty- or a hundred-fold would be impossible aerobically. You would have to pump around fifty to a hundred times more blood. You'd have to have a huge heart."

To this day no one really knows how quickly muscle fibers contract in a human being, or even in a laboratory animal. There have been countless experiments in which scientists studied muscle in the laboratory, electrically stimulating the tissue to see how fast it can contract. Fast-twitch fibers take about 50 milliseconds to reach their peak tension when stimulated, whereas slow-twitch fibers take about 110 milliseconds. But, according to Rome, when scientists study mammals in the laboratory, they are looking at a mixture of fiber types, even in muscle that appears to be predominantly of one type. And when that muscle is used, the body turns to the fiber it needs for a particular task. If you are walking, for example, your quadriceps muscle (in front of your thigh) will use its slow-twitch fibers, even though it also has fast-twitch ones.

Another complication when muscle is studied in the laboratory comes from the trade-off in muscle between the speed with which muscle contracts and the power it generates. The faster it contracts, the less power, Rome says, explaining that it is the same principle as the one that governs speed and power when you ride a bike. You can put a bike in the lowest gear and spin the wheels very fast, but you will not generate much power. Or you can switch to the highest gear, and generate a lot of power, but you will not have much speed.

But precise measurements of muscle speed and force, and the distinctions between fast- and slow-twitch muscles, are impossible in the case of mammals. And even with amphibians, the insights are recent. Rome's work began with a paper he published in 1988. "It was the first time anyone had taken muscles out and measured their speed in relation to their function in the body," Rome says.

But, I ask, what about the dogma that sprinters have more fast-twitch muscle and distance runners have more slow-twitch muscle? I had thought that was established by biopsy studies of athletes, taking tiny portions of their muscle and analyzing it. Rome tells me that it would not surprise him if the conclusions were correct, and the repeated measurements of each athlete's muscle adds a bit more credibility to the conclusions. But the biopsies cannot determine incontrovertibly a person's predominant muscle type. "When they do muscle biopsies, they take one-tenth of one-hundredth of one percent of a muscle," he says. "We have to hope that that's representative of the muscle. But there are well-known differences in the distribution of fiber types between muscles and within muscles. When these guys say fast-twitch muscles are used for sprinting and slow-twitch are used for jogging, that's never been measured in a really direct way."

If you train to become fast, doing sprints, for example, you would want to have as much fast-twitch muscle as possible. That gives rise to another question: If you force a white muscle to work like a red one, will it turn into a red muscle? And then, if you can convert muscle, will performance change?

The same question also relates to aging. As people grow old, they appear to lose muscle in general, but fast-twitch muscles in particular. Is that why old people are so slow? And can this aging process be slowed, or even prevented, with training?

When the work began in the 1960s, scientists thought that muscles were immutable and that, if anything, the muscles determined how the nerve cells that were attached to them behaved. A nerve attached to a fast-twitch muscle conducts intermittent, high-frequency bursts of impulses; one attached to a slow-twitch muscle conducts more continuous trains of impulses, and at a lower frequency. Scientists thought that these firing characteristics were determined by chemicals that traveled from the muscle fibers to the nerve cells. They devised a test of that hypothesis—they would hook a slow nerve to a fast-twitch muscle and ask: Do the corresponding nerve cells acquire the characteristics of fast-firing nerves? And will the opposite happen if they hook a fast nerve to a slow-twitch muscle?

The results were a surprise. It turned out that the nerve cells did not change, although the muscles did. A slow nerve changed fast-twitch muscles into slow-twitch ones, converting much of the tangled mix of fast- and slow-twitch fibers into a muscle that was essentially of one type, the slow-twitch red muscle. And the opposite happened when fast-twitch nerves were hooked to muscles that consisted predominantly of slow-twitch fibers. The influence seemed to be from nerve to muscle, rather than from muscle to nerve.

"This was a very important experiment," said Stanley Salmons, a muscle researcher at the University of Liverpool in England. "It showed that a muscle isn't the type it is forever." He wondered, however, about the proposed explanation for the effect. Scientists hypothesized that an unidentified chemical or hormone diffused down the nerve and into the muscle, changing its properties. Why not propose that the nerve's electrical impulse was the crucial factor, asked Salmons. He found a way to test that alternate hypothesis.

"I was a postgraduate fellow at the time at the University of Birmingham, and I was building an electrical circuit for something else," he says. "By chance, I discovered a circuit that was hardly taking any current. I realized what I could use it for." He could stimulate a muscle purely with electricity, while not changing the nerve at all. That would eliminate any possibility of a hormone or other chemical diffusing down a nerve to alter a muscle. And if the muscle still changed, he would have proved it was the nature of the electrical activity that did it.

While the experiment sounds obvious, Salmons says that back in the 1960s it seemed an impossible undertaking, simply because scientists had not developed the devices they needed for such an experiment—stimulators that could be completely implanted in small laboratory animals and that could last for the many weeks required of such an experiment. His device changed all that.

When he did the critical experiment, using the pale, predominantly fast-twitch leg muscles from a rabbit and stimulating them with pulses of electricity like those from a slow-twitch nerve, it worked, and it worked astonishingly well. The muscle fibers turned red, converting from fast- to slow-twitch. To him, the conclusion was obvious: muscle can change from one type to another, depending on the electrical impulses it receives. No mysterious chemicals or hormones need be invoked. But others were not convinced.

"In those days, people didn't believe me. I had quite a fight on my hands," Salmons says. "The team that did the cross-innervation was headed by Jack Eccles, a Nobel Prize winner, so people would pay attention to him. I was just a Ph.D. student."

So he did another experiment. First, he took fast muscles and stimulated them for five months with a slow type of impulse pattern. They became even slower than the natural so-called slow muscles—a much bigger effect than had ever been seen with cross-innervation. Then he took slow muscles and hooked them up to fast nerves, but he stimulated half of them electrically as if they were slow nerves. The muscles that only received fast nerves became faster, but the ones that received the slow pattern of activity as well did not change, remaining slow-twitch. If you changed the activity but didn't change the nerve, the muscle altered its type. If you changed the nerve but didn't change the activity, the muscle didn't alter. Activity, not the nerve, had to be the factor responsible.

"That paper, published in *Nature* in 1976, was the nail in the coffin of the chemical theory," Salmons says. Finally, scientists believed him. "There are one or two people around who still believe the old idea, but it's literally one or two," Salmons tells me.

Exercise is the same, in principle, as electrical stimulation, he adds, but it involves less of the muscle, and the stimulation is for less time. With exercise the main changes are in the muscle's metabolism, rather than the speed it contracts. When someone trains to run a marathon, they are stimulating leg muscles to develop endurance rather than explosive power. Those adaptations can make the difference between being able to finish the race and breaking down in exhaustion. "Through daily training for long periods, you can get the sort of muscles that a marathoner has," Salmons says. And if you train like a sprinter? Your muscles will develop a greater proportion of pale, fast-twitch fibers, he adds.

Then why not simply train by hooking your muscles to an electric current? Why go through the agony of long, grueling sessions on a track or running for mile after mile on the road? The problems are practical ones.

"If you stimulate with surface electrodes on the skin, it is impossibly painful to get all the muscle stimulated," Salmons says. "The danger is that people will put on these stimulators and they will stimulate the surface fibers but not the deep fibers. If you then imagine a fatigue situation—you go out running and part of the muscle fatigues and the rest doesn't—that could be quite damaging. The other way to do it is to put the wires inside the muscle. But then you do so much damage that it's not a good idea either. In any case, sports performance is about more than just training individual muscles. You are training coordination between muscles, and developing your heart and lungs, too."

Scientists still do not know exactly how the muscle changes take place. They know that there are signals that alter protein production in muscle cells and that those signals switch genes on and off. But, says Salmons, "we know very little about what those signals are."

I tell Cynthia about training. We're sitting on wrought-iron chairs on a small bluestone patio in her backyard. It is a breezy summer day and she is complaining that she never seems to get any stronger. She has been working out, on a sporadic basis, with a personal trainer at her gym, but even though she has been a gym member for years, she looks just the same and is no stronger, no more fit. She walks in the neighborhood, as always, but she is no faster and still gets slightly out of breath if she tries to walk quickly up a long shallow hill. But is the problem that her trainer is incompetent? Or that Cynthia works out inconsistently? Or that she is not pushing herself? Or is it none of these? Could it be that Cynthia's body, for whatever reason, is not trainable?

"Everyone can train," says Anna Hess, the Spinning instructor and personal trainer at my gym. It is the end of one of her classes and we are wiping down our bikes. Anna is matter-of-factly noting that some people come to Spinning classes week after week, faithfully showing up after work or on weekends, and they never get any better. But that, she says, is because they put no effort into the class. They keep the resistance on their pedals low, they pay no attention to their heart rates, they barely sweat—and so, of course, their bodies never change. But, she insists, anyone who tries, anyone who puts effort into it, can and will get better. Their bodies will be trained.

Exercise physiologists used to think that way too, Costill tells me. When people said they were training and their endurance never got better, it was assumed that those people were dissembling or deluding themselves. Scientists viewed these exercisers like many view overweight people who swear they are always on a diet.

The truth about training gradually emerged when a scientist, Claude Bouchard, who had spent his career studying fat people, decided to put the training hypothesis to a test. What would happen, he asked, if he had people train in an exercise laboratory, where he could watch them and see for himself whether they really were working? It would be the exercise equivalent of obesity experiments (such as Pete Ahrens's study) that put people into metabolic research units of hospitals and measured exactly what they ate and how many calories they burned and how much they weighed.

Around 1980, he began a series of studies, working at Lavalle

University in Quebec. His work attracted little attention at first. He was attempting mainly to satisfy his own curiosity with regard to issues that grew out of his work as an obesity researcher. He had seen fat person after fat person and had discovered that there is a strong genetic component to obesity. Identical twins tend to have nearly identical weights; fat parents have fat children; thin people who agree to gain weight for the sake of science, eating so much each day that they feel vaguely ill, quickly and effortlessly drop back down to their original weights as soon as the study is over. Could there also be a genetic component to fitness, Bouchard wondered. Were there people who were out of shape and who would never be fit? They might be like the fat people who are doomed to be obese because some genetically determined balance of chemicals in their bodies drives them to eat enough to maintain a very high weight. Bouchard decided that he had seen enough in his research to make it worthwhile to investigate fitness as he had investigated obesity.

"I asked the question because I had seen people who were known as couch potatoes," Bouchard tells me. "They were very sedentary, but when we measured them, there were quite a lot of differences among them. Some had a very nice cardiorespiratory endurance, and at the other end of the spectrum there were people who were very deteriorated from a fitness point of view. I said, 'Maybe this problem is caused by genetic differences. Maybe there are also differences in the way they respond to fitness programs.' I decided to base a whole research program on that."

The first study began in 1982, with a call for men and women aged 18 to 30 who were totally inactive, with a lifetime history of being almost completely sedentary, but who were not particularly fat. The scientists did not want to confuse inactivity due to obesity with inactivity due to a possible genetic tendency to being averse to any physical exercise. When they advertised for subjects, they found them, 129 men and women who were extremely inactive. From them, Bouchard says, "we picked thirty who were at the bottom of the pile—really, really sedentary. We questioned them and we measured their activity in the last weeks, months, and year. They had desk jobs, they would drive a car and never walk. They never did any sport."

For twenty weeks, these volunteers came to the lab for physical training. "It was a very standardized program, everyone did the same things in the lab so we could not say that some were not compliant." They would walk on a treadmill and ride a stationary bike. "They began at 30 minutes a day, four days a week. Then they moved up to five days a week, up to 50 minutes a day, up to an intensity of 85 percent of their maximum heart rate. These guys discovered that they could exercise." But their physiological responses were very different. "We had large differences in respiration, in maximum oxygen uptake, in the results of muscle and adipose tissue biopsies," says Bouchard, referring to changes in endurance and the ability to exercise at a high intensity as well as changes in body fat and the size of different types of muscle fibers. "Some did not gain in fitness. Others improved by 50 percent, 60 percent. But they were all compliant."

That, he says, suggested that genetic differences in responses to training do exist.

Next, he did a study with interval training. Once again, the subjects were truly sedentary and once again they did all of their workouts in the lab. "We found the same thing," Bouchard says. "Some responded and some did not."

To see if these differences were caused by genetic variations, he did the studies again with pairs of identical twins. "We found the same thing—high responders and low responders," he noted. But, predictably, however one twin of a pair responded, the other twin did, too. "Some were high responders, some were low responders, and some were late responders," Bouchard reports. The stage was set, he tells me, to begin an effort to find the actual genes that determine if someone can be trained, and if so, how much. Bouchard now heads the Pennington Biomedical Research Center at Louisiana State University, where he directs five research centers in the project: at Pennington, Washington University in St. Louis, Indiana University, Texas A&M, and the University of Minnesota. The investigators recruited 100 white families and 100 black families, for a total of 742 subjects. All the children were 17 and older, so they, too, were subjects in the study.

"We tested, trained, and retested them with the same program," Bouchard says. And we have found the same thing in each of the clinical centers. There are high responders and low responders." One measurement of a training response is the increase in the amount of oxygen people use when they try to push themselves hard. The average increase after training was 400 milliliters of oxygen. But the range was zero milliliters to 1,000 milliliters. The standard deviation was 200, meaning that about two-thirds of the people increased their oxygen consumption by 200 to 600 milliliters of oxygen.

"These are huge differences," Bouchard explains. "But within families you have aggregation." Children tend to respond the way their parents do. Siblings tend to respond like each other. The heritability of responsiveness to exercise training was at least as great as it is for body weight, blood pressure, and cholesterol, Bouchard tells me.

It also turned out that despite a popular belief that people who exercise regularly will substantially increase their levels of HDL, the protein that protects against heart disease, the actual improvement is minimal. One analysis of fifty-nine studies found that the average rise on HDL was only two points. Bouchard found that the increase was about 2 percent or less, unless the people also lost weight. And in those cases, Bouchard found that the improvement was really due to weight loss.

Bouchard's group has no immediate plans to reveal to its test participants what their genes reveal about their ability to exercise. But, he says, he knows from all the work so far that some people, about 10 percent of the population, really will never get any better with exercise, their endurance will never improve, they will never get faster, and they will never get stronger. He personally has given some people that grim prognosis. These were people, he says, who probably knew what was happening. "They did not improve their endurance. They did not lose a gram of fat," Bouchard says. These are people who may simply give up on exercise, and understandably. While they may still derive some health benefits from exercise, the tenuous promise of possibly improved health may be a hard sell for people who may want to look better or feel more vigorous. How many years can people go on with no outward signs of improvement? "That may be the reason some people abandon exercise," Bouchard concludes.

What if you want to train but are a nonresponder? "If you can monitor things beyond your performance, you may find good reasons to exercise," Bouchard says. "If not, you have to be convinced that exercise does something good for you, even though you will be the last one to finish each race."

The good news, however, is that most people do respond, and some, about 10 percent, respond astonishingly well. I had a feeling that anyone who signed up for Mount Everest already had some indication that their body could be trained. We, after all, were the exercise zealots, and I doubt we would like exercise so much if we never improved.

The Mount Everest ride, of course, was not a serious athletic competition, and compared to feats like a 100-kilometer run it seemed almost pitiful. But I have the same feeling that Bernd Heinrich must have had—I was going to have to change my body if I was to do it well. And the more I learn about the eccentricities of athletes and trainers, the more I wonder about who was behind this ride and the training program that Bill and I were following.

six

THE ATHLETE'S WORLD

The Mount Everest ride is going to take place at Evolutions Fitness, a gym I had never heard of before, and for good reason. It is not part of a chain, it has no large signs directing one to it, and it is a half-hour drive from my house, when the traffic is not backed up.

"Evolutions?" asks Sam Bruno. "That little place in East Windsor?" When I see it, I know what he means. It is at one end of a drab strip mall in a sprawling town in central New Jersey. At the other end of the mall is the yellow symbol of what many Europeans and the self-righteously healthy everywhere hate most about America: the golden arches of McDonald's, which perfumes the air with the unmistakable aroma of fried food. On Friday nights, the line to the drive-up window is clogged with cars.

Evolutions is, in every way, the opposite of the McDonald's mentality. It is a gym that, despite its futuristic name, looks like a health club that failed to evolve, a throwback to the days when gyms were low-rent affairs peopled by tattooed bodybuilders grunting loudly as they hoisted huge barbells loaded with heavy weights and guzzling protein shakes on their way out the door.

You enter Evolutions through a short narrow hallway that delivers you to a space looking onto the gym's three cement-floored rooms. To your right is a weight-lifting room, with its obligatory rubber floor covering. Black-and-chrome bodybuilding machines are next to racks of free weights and benches to sit or lie on while lifting barbells and dumbbells. In the back is a barren baby-sitting room facing the Dumpsters in the rear parking lot. And to your left is a large square room for exercise classes, with a floor painted slate blue and with plate-glass windows that look out on the parking lot and highway in front of the gym. There are no lockers and the men's and women's dressing rooms are cramped, no-nonsense affairs, each with a single sink and toilet, a couple of small showers, and a small wooden bench. No one lingers in them and few stop to preen under the unforgiving light cast by a bulb in the ceiling.

But the gym's owner is not a former champion bodybuilder with a huge chest and powerful thighs. Instead, it is Sharon, a forty-one-year-old with slim hips, shoulder-length honey-blond hair, and a turned-up nose, looking like an advertiser's notion of the all-American woman in the mid-1970s. She is an unlikely businesswoman—she never went to college and almost stumbled into owning a gym—but she single-handedly turned Evolutions into a central New Jersey Spinning attraction.

Sharon was a gymnast when she was a teenager but did not do well in meets because of stage fright. After high school, she became a dental technician, choosing that job "because they were willing to train someone." She worked her way up to managing a dentist's office. Then, eight years after graduating from high school, after marriage and three children, she tired of the long hours and began teaching at a gymnastics school. There she met another young woman who was an aerobics instructor at Evolutions and who told Sharon that the gym was run down and struggling financially. Sharon decided to buy it and make it into her vision of what a gym should be.

"I never liked walking into the latest gyms. I always felt intimidated," she says. "I felt like I had to be at a certain fitness level. I wanted a gym where people would just come in and work out, where it was friendly." No need to dress up to display one's tight, muscular body. And she did not want to force her clients to sign long-term contracts, something she thinks has driven people away from gym memberships.

She sought out exercise instructors who would make novices feel comfortable; she ended up dismissing some who did not meet that standard. "I had some instructors who were prima donnas. They put themselves above the members," she explains. She chose not to install television sets, deciding that nothing is more boring than walking on a treadmill and watching TV. And she told members that she had no interest in knowing their body-fat composition or how much they weighed. At her insistence, there are no scales at Evolutions.

Some members looked askance. "I had one woman who said, 'How come you don't weigh people? How come you don't measure them?' I told her that I have no control over what you do when you leave the gym," Sharon said.

At the same time, Sharon began running, longer and longer distances, and discovered that she loved exercise that depended on endurance. "The longer I went, the more fun I had. A one-mile run eventually turned into fourteen miles." Then she discovered Spinning, became certified as a Spinning instructor, and bought ten of the special stationary bikes for her gym. Soon she was obsessed with the sport, teaching thirteen, fourteen classes a week. "I began to understand that it is very easy to get addicted," Sharon says.

She learned that the inventor of Spinning, a former competitive cyclist from Australia named Johnny G (for Goldberg) was going to lead a twelve-hour Spinning ride in Culver City, California, and she told Kathryn Schwartz and another Spinning instructor at her gym, Sue Barnhart.

"I said I've got to go. I can't not go," Sharon related. "They were, like, 'Why?' And I told them, 'Never again will you be able to ride twelve hours with Johnny G.' Somehow they were convinced." Kathryn and Sue were persuaded—they would go with her—but others thought she had lost her mind. Her friends told her she was crazy to pay $500 to go all the way across the country to sit on a bike in a gym and pedal for twelve hours. Sharon had a different opinion. "It was the chance of a lifetime."

Part of it was an opportunity to meet and ride with Johnny G, a legendary figure in the fitness culture. He had a way of talking about exercise that took it beyond the exercise-as-medicine, walk-to-help-your-heart level. For Johnny G, pushing yourself, testing your limits, was a spiritual experience. Sharon knew the outlines of his story—it was legend among Spinning enthusiasts, and, like others, she found it inspirational.

Johnny got the idea for Spinning after a dreadful attempt in 1994 to compete in the Race Across America, a nonstop cross-country bicycle race from Los Angeles to New York City. To win it, you can't waste time resting, or even sleeping, and riders tell of hallucinating from fatigue and sleep deprivation. For Johnny G, the shock was that none of his extensive training had prepared him for the ride.

He recalled those awful days of the race: "I think it must be like taking a birthing class and you think you have everything you need—until the labor pains kick in. Nothing could have prepared me for the spasms of my calves, the flesh ripping away from the seams of my cycling shorts on the back of my thighs and my butt, the sweat pouring down my arms like I'm a salty waterfall, while parts of myself drop along the road, skin and sweat and brain cells falling away."

He was in a haze. "I vaguely remember riding through sleeping towns in the middle of the night, passing dark houses with families warm in their bed." And he knew the tricks the mind can play. "A fellow rider told me that once during the RAAM, after being on the road for a week, he started thinking his crew members were aliens who were trying to possess his body. He got so freaked out, he drove off the road and wouldn't take any food because he thought they were trying to poison him."

"So why am I doing this?" Johnny wrote in a memoir. "Better

not to ponder that one. 'Why?' is a bad question, a dangerous tributary to follow . . . But there has to be a reason here beside my desire to arrive at the finish line as one of the greatest ultra-distance cyclists of all time."

In Indianapolis, six days and 2,000 miles from Los Angeles, 400 miles from the finish line, his resolve began to waver.

"Satan says I have to pedal until I drop because I can't let down my sponsors. And what about all the people who didn't offer me any support? He says I have to show them what I'm made of, so they'll respect me."

"Christ says I need to make a choice for myself. He says true strength isn't necessarily about finishing. It's also about walking away with my consciousness intact. He says no one can ever take this race away from me because I'll be quitting of my own accord."

He stopped and got off his bike, stunning the leader of his crew, who were riding along in a car to support him. Johnny returned to California to reexamine his life. He realized that despite the agony and the pain, the endless training and even the shock of riding the Race Across America, his life as an athlete had been a great gift.

"When an athlete learns to face adversity with maximum effort, there is a good chance to be victorious," he notes. "All athletes must accept the fact that if you're not hurting, you're not going hard enough, but whether the output feels hard or easy is not the point. The point of the game is mastery of self-confrontation. It's about continuing to press forward, to go with the flow of the energy and to be the best that you can be, no matter the physical obstacles or the voices screaming in your head. I have found that without exerting enough effort to go into the depths of what life has to offer, I'm not going to uncover the treasure within."

Johnny decided to find a way for ordinary people to experience what he had felt on a bike. He thought that they could do it in a gym, but not with ordinary stationary bikes, which, he decided, were never going to be suitable. Instead, he remembered rollers, a device for indoor bicycling that had been popular among serious bicyclists, who used it for off-season training in the 1970s and eighties.

I know this device well—Bill and I used to have one. We rode it in a tiny apartment when we were students, installing it in a doorframe. We rode it in our garage when we got our first house. When Johnny says, "It takes absolute dedication and concentration to remain upright," I can only agree.

Rollers are actually metal cylinders, fifteen inches long and a few inches in diameter, supported by a metal frame. Johnny aptly describes the device as "three very slippery drums (two at the back and one in front)." You would balance your bike on the rollers and pedal furiously. If you stop or even slow down, your bike falls over—and you quickly reach out for a nearby wall to keep from toppling to the ground. That was why we put our device in a doorframe. If you ride too fast, you can ride off the end of the rollers and crash. The same can happen if you are not completely balanced while riding. Bill got used to the rollers, but I never did; to me, they were always terrifying. Johnny thought back on them in 1994, when he was looking for a way to give ordinary people the experience of riding like a bike racer. The rollers led him to build a hand-welded prototype of a Spinning bike. Of course, there is no problem balancing on a Spinning bike—the frame keeps the bike erect. But the front wheel is something like the front cylinder of the rollers, spinning away as you pedal.

"The stationary bike would no longer exist solely for warming up or for burning calories before training," Johnny wrote. "It would now be an entire workout unto itself, on a functional piece of equipment with real handlebars, a water-bottle cage and a variety of settings that offered the ability to emulate everything a cyclist did on the road—time trials, riding the flats, climbing a mountain, maneuvering bumps in the road, sprinting—in a single forty-minute session.

"The playing field is level," he says. Each person in the room is working at his or her own level, challenging themselves. "You have to find your own limit."

He elaborated in a memoir: "Even if you choose never to see the starting line of an actual race or deal with the winds, the deserts, the mountains, and the leg cramps, I can show you how to liberate yourself through the Spinning program. I can show you what it feels like to be in the middle or the front of the pack without suffering the humiliation of being dropped from the team because you aren't good enough."

"For forty minutes, three times a week, I'm going to make you think, believe, and feel like a real human being. You will find the pedal strokes to take you to the top of the hill.

"My goal for the Spinning program was to inspire nobility of spirit."

For Sharon, there could be no greater experience than a ride with the master himself, Johnny G. If any ride could be transforming, it would be this one.

She, Kathryn, and Sue knew they had to train, so they began making up a program as they went along. They decided that if they were to ride for twelve hours, they would have to first endure eight hours on the bikes at Evolutions.

They trained at the gym in the middle of the day in the middle of the week, when few clients were there, riding for hours on end. They hoisted themselves onto the Spinning bikes in the exercise room and started to pedal, playing music, grabbing bottles of water from a cooler they kept on the floor next to them, eating fruits and special exercise foods—sports bars and sports gels and sports drinks. Sharon recalls the day she did her eight-hour training ride. She set up her Spinning bike beside the desk where clients signed in, climbed up on it, and began pedaling.

"I had some food, I had some water, and I would do certain things. I would say, 'Okay, I'm going to do ten minutes of a seated climb and ten minutes of a standing run and ten minutes of jumps.' And the thing that is so amazing is that while that was probably the most fit that I had ever been, it wasn't the physical part of it that was hard. It was the mental. I could not even fathom riding for twelve hours. And as I'm sitting here today, I say to myself, 'Why did I ever want to do that?' "

The twelve-hour ride with Johnny G? "It was bizarre. There was actually a wedding ceremony in the middle of it. A Spinning instructor from Germany and a Spinning instructor from South Africa who met through Spinning got married. They had rose petals all over the place and they had a priest come in who performed the ceremony. During that time, we had to sit on the bikes but we couldn't ride."

Sharon took a break every hour and changed her clothes twice during the ride. She ate the food that assistants brought to her, drank lots of water, and ate salt when it was offered to her. "I never thought in my life that I would eat straight table salt and enjoy it," she says. "You'd wet your fingers, put them in the salt, and eat it."

For her, the twelve-hour ride was neither fun nor even exhilarating. And Johnny G did not lead the group the way that Spinning instructors usually do, talking, inspiring, coaching, and generally prodding a room full of exercisers to work harder than they could on their own. Instead, he seemed sometimes to be in his own world, manic or withdrawn, making odd demands. Ten hours into the ride, he told everyone to get off the bikes and go outside and breathe the fresh air. Yet the room was already open to the outside and fresh air was not a problem. Sharon recalls that when she stepped outside with the others, she came close to losing her resolve—how hard it was to go back in and climb back on her bike!

But the Johnny G ride gave her the idea to try special events, rides that did not fit into the typical Spinning curriculum, that would require special training and dedication, and that would give members at her gym goals to aim for. Her first event, she decided, would mark the millennium—two thousand jumps for the year 2000. A jump is a Spinning move that involves standing up, then sitting down again, pedaling all the while. It is tiring, a motion that is guaranteed to make your heart rate climb, and it is not a move that road bicyclists do. Those Spinning enthusiasts who decided to accept this challenge trained, of course, doing repeated jumps in Spinning classes. Sharon would hold classes in which the group would do nothing but jumps.

The goal for New Year's Day of the year 2000 was to do the jumps within three hours, but the group of seventeen devotees completed the jumps in 2 hours and 40 minutes, Sharon says. Somehow, with what seems like a hit-or-miss approach, the group had trained, and their training had worked.

The next year, she was approached by Josh Taylor, one of Johnny G's "master presenters," who told her he had an idea for a new kind of Spinning event. He called it Mount Everest.

Mount Everest was Josh Taylor's dream and inspiration, his way of conveying the thrill of competition to a group of people who might never have known it except vicariously. He is twenty-eight but looks younger, six feet one, but he looks taller. Josh is all arms and legs, long and lean with short, ice-blond hair, a narrow Nordic face. When he teaches a Spinning class, he has a way of chuckling demonically, "*Heh heh heh . . .*" as he asks you to push yourself a little harder. He tips his head far back and squirts water from his water bottle down his throat, then tells his class to remember to drink. He has a midwestern aw-shucks air about him and a surfer dude's use of language.

Josh, like Johnny before he invented Spinning, is part of a world that is hidden from most of us. I think of it as a parallel world of athletics. It is made up of those whose job it is to exercise, to train, to be fit. And it is a world that is completely separate from the world of people like Bill, Cynthia, or me, people who work in offices all day, or who spend their days at home doing volunteer work and chauffeuring children and going to meetings of the Garden Club. Yet Josh, in planning Mount Everest, was trying to give us a glimpse of that other life and a chance to experience some aspects of it for ourselves.

We can never really live the lives of its year-round inhabitants, of course, but Josh hoped to show us that we can do more than just read about athletes or watch their exploits. He wanted to let us actually feel some of the emotions and rewards that drive people like him, and to feel the extraordinary changes in the body's physiology that can occur when you push yourself hard—if, that is, you are genetically able to train. For just a brief time, he thought, we might be able to see his world.

When I think of the parallel world of athletes like Josh and his attempts to reveal it to the Mount Everest riders, I think of a phrase used by Bob Massie. Bob is now the executive director of Ceres, a coalition of environmental, investment, and advocacy groups that is based in Boston. He is a natural diplomat with a warm smile and a handsome bearded face, and a body that is subtly crippled by hemophilia, a genetic disease. When he was born, his medical problems were a complete surprise. No one in his family had ever had hemophilia, and his parents, Robert and Suzanne Massie, knew little about it. They ended up writing a book, *Journey*, about their efforts to raise a disabled child whose medical crises were unpredictable and unrelenting.

When he was college age, Bob contributed to a chapter in his parents' book, describing what it was like to be a person with a gravely serious genetic disorder. Articulate, intelligent, educated, he thought of himself as "bridging the gap," poised between the disabled, who were unable to speak for themselves, and the healthy, who had no idea of what life was like for those with a chronic disease. His role, he said, was to speak for those who never were heard.

Of course, what Bob Massie went through was transforming and excruciating in a way that makes it seem as if one is almost trivializing his experience to use his phrase in another context. He wrote about the contrast between watching the swimming team practice at Harvard and thinking of a little boy, Jamie, he had met in Los Angeles who had a genetic disease that made him so fragile that his bones were constantly breaking.

"I would think of Jamie as he swam and then I would think of the Harvard guys as they swam, and I would think of myself as I swam. I realized that the Harvard men would feel nothing but pity for Jamie, and Jamie would not understand the Harvard men at all. But, amazingly, I felt at home with both kinds of people and yet somehow was not in either place.

"And suddenly, I had a revelation," he continued. "I saw myself as bridging the gap. So when I would get tired, I'd think, 'You're bridging the gap. You've got to work harder.' "

In a way, what Josh was doing was letting some of us bridge a different gap, the gap between the athletes who have an inborn talent, a fluke of the genetic shuffle, that sets them apart from almost everyone else on earth, and the ordinary people who have never trained, never challenged themselves, never asked what their bodies were capable of doing. I remembered Bob Massie's words and I thought that Josh was giving us a gift, by letting us into his world.

Athletes are born to excel, with a talent every bit as rare as a high IQ. And, like the opera star who only by chance discovers she can sing, many athletes, like Josh, say it was purely fortuitous that they discovered the sport they were born for.

Dave Costill, the exercise physiologist at Ball State, tells me he often muses on the athletes that might have been. They are physical geniuses, in a way, and could easily fall by the wayside if they never tried their sport. He thinks about the thousands, or millions, of people in the world with extraordinarily high IQs who never know it and who never got an education. And he thinks about the athletes he discovered, by accident, who turned out to be stars.

When Costill was first starting out, at the State University of New York at Cortland, he decided to look for new talent for the cross-country team. He put out a call for all students who had any sort of running background or who might want to try the sport. In the end, he recruited fifteen young men—of whom three were so good they made All-American that year. They were first, second, and third in every meet in 1964. Cortland's yearbook that year states, "It got to the point that they were calling three of the runners 'The Untouchables.' " Yet none had previously had any inkling they were so gifted.

One had been a high school runner, but his distance was a mile, not the five miles of a college cross-country event. Another was a muscular ex–football player. And the third was Bob Fitts, who simply decided he needed a sport. "He turned out to be the best," Costill says. He was so good that in a race against Syracuse he set a record that stood for twenty-five years. In 1996, Cortland inducted Fitts into its Athletic Hall of Fame, hailing him as "the greatest male distance runner in SUNY Cortland history."

Fitts used to argue with Costill that anyone could be a champion if they tried hard enough. But eventually, Costill relates, Fitts conceded that genetics might possibly have something to do with it.

Yet the classic story of discovering hidden talent was Costill's experience with bicyclists. One day not long after he had come to Ball State, where he was directing the Human Performance Laboratory and teaching, Costill made a chance remark to a graduate-level physiology class. He observed that the local bicycling team was training incorrectly for an upcoming event. Instead of pushing themselves with intervals and endurance rides, they were just going out and riding. "I said I bet I could take those guys and train them so they would win the race."

One of the students in the class, Edmund Burke, was a bicyclist himself and decided to take Costill up on the offer. "He came up after class and said, 'I've got a team for you. Try to train us.' " Burke then recruited some of his fraternity brothers, among them his roommate, Tom Doughty.

It was a type of race that is rarely seen outside of bicycling.

The goal was to go eighty times around a track. Each team puts one rider in the race. That person rides for a while and then, typically, the coach will put in someone else to continue. It does not matter how many or how few of the team's members get to ride— all that matters is to have your team's rider be first to finish the race.

Doughty, who had never even thought about bicycle racing, turned out to be so much better than anyone else on the team that no one could ride with him. Finally, it was the day of the race, a time to see if Costill's training had made a difference. Doughty was the first rider from his team to hit the track, cycling furiously and tirelessly, around and around for sixty laps. By then, the others on the team were chafing, wanting their own chance to ride, so Doughty pulled over. Soon, his team, which had been far ahead of the competition, was falling behind. Doughty got back on his bike, rode the last few laps, and won the race for the team.

He went on to become a national champion in individual and team trial races and qualified for the 1980 U.S. Olympic bicycling team.

Josh Taylor discovered his talent when he was a bit younger, in high school, when he happened to go on a bike ride with a friend. He was growing up in Quakertown, Pennsylvania, a small town about forty miles north of Philadelphia. No one in his family was particularly athletic; his parents encouraged him, but they, like his three sisters, were indifferent to sports. He knew he had athletic talent because he was a gifted volleyball player, so good that he even made the National Junior Olympics team. But he never felt an all-consuming passion for volleyball and he never felt it was something beyond a high school activity.

One day, when Josh was in ninth grade, a friend loaned him his father's old Schwinn bike and took him out on a twenty-mile ride on the country roads outside of town. Immediately Josh was hooked. It was as though he had found his calling.

"We went tearing down the road and I thought it was the

coolest thing in the world. I was like, 'This is awesome,' " he said. He started saving his money to buy a bike of his own, and soon he was out on the road, alone, riding thirty or forty miles every day, riding before volleyball practice, dreaming of riding when he sat in his high school classes, absolutely obsessed with the sport.

He discovered that not far away was the Lehigh Valley Velodrome, a track made for bicycle racing. Velodrome tracks, with their banked sides, look like miniature versions of NASCAR tracks. Josh showed up and was enthralled. "They had a program there with national-level coaches helping people who had never done racing." He became a star, winning a fifteen-lap race so dramatically that he was a lap ahead of his nearest competitor. The riders were divided into an A group and a B group. Josh was an A. By then he was in eleventh grade. None of his friends raced— they simply shrugged at his passion. "My friends were all, 'Okay. Whatever, dude.' "

Soon Josh was getting friendly with some of the professional racers he met at the velodrome and he began training with them. When he graduated from high school, he enrolled in a small community college near his home, but his heart was not in academics.

"I was, like, 'You know what, I'm really digging the cycling thing,' " Josh says. "So I pulled out of school and pursued it full time."

He was so good that he rose through the cycling categories in leaps, like skipping grades in school. First he was a junior cyclist, in category 5, the lowest. Soon he was promoted directly to category 2 because he was so fast, and within a year he was category 1, the best.

Bicycle racing is a grueling sport. "It's probably the hardest sport to be good at," Josh says. "You spend six or seven hours a day training, building an endurance base, because you have to be able to go really hard. Then you go home and you're so wasted from training. But you've got to eat right, you have to sleep right, you've got to get a massage. If you want to be at the top, there's just no backing down. It's your entire life."

It is a life with rewards that can come only sporadically. Sometimes he wins a race, sometimes a big one, like the Pennsylvania State Pro Racing Championship, which he won twice. But then there are all those races he did not win, and all that training and effort that can seem for naught.

"The times are just so few and far between when you do really well that they're just huge to you," Josh tells me. The bicycling season begins in March and continues through the end of September, with races across the country involving 100 to 150 cyclists.

Money is tight. Racers need sponsors, but few companies want to invest in athletes who compete in a sport that is so far from the public eye. "It's tough—a lot of the big companies are looking for TV coverage, but how much of cycling is on TV?" Josh asks. He got lucky, signing up with Zone Perfect, a company that makes energy bars. He loves the product, he insists, but quickly offers to send me a case, remarking that he's gotten a little tired of eating them. For his pay, he is supposed to actively promote the company.

"You do appearances. I write articles for Zone Perfect's Web site," Josh says. It also helps that his wife, Julie, who was his childhood sweetheart, has a good job, running a corporate fitness center for employees of Johnson & Johnson, the drug company.

On a typical day, Josh wakes up at eight a.m., after sleeping for nine hours. He eats a huge breakfast of eggs, toast, a couple of bowls of cereal, and a protein shake made with a banana and Zone Perfect whey soy protein, a supplement powder that the Zone Perfect company alleges has all the necessary protein building blocks. By nine a.m., he is on the road, bicycling to the velodrome for his training. It takes him thirty-five to forty minutes to get there on the country roads. He rides hard all day at the track, working with his trainer and fellow cyclists.

I ask him why he does it, what the motivation is for such a grueling and spartan existence. He lives, he says, for those moments when his exertion is so great that he experiences an almost out-of-body sensation. He tries to explain.

"It's living at the extreme edge of life, pushing yourself to the very edge," Josh tells me. "You're just suffering. Why do I put myself through it? You're just living . . . you're just fully living. Nothing much matters, but every breath and every muscle in your body is telling you to stop."

He pauses, grasping for words. "Maybe it's not just the physical side, maybe it's the mental side. I wish I could write down what I feel. You're at the edge of living. You're *right there*. You're pushing yourself to the limit. A friend of mine says it's like going into space. You worked so hard to get out of the earth's gravity and now it's so beautiful. You're floating. You're not supposed to be there and you can only be there for a short amount of time. But when you come off it you're, like, 'That was pretty cool.' "

Josh seems an unlikely person to lead a group Spinning ride. He spends his days with other athletes. All his friends are in that parallel world. Why, I ask, would he care about people like us?

He says he discovered Spinning a few years ago, by chance, and for many of the same reasons that my husband Bill took up the sport. He was lifting weights on a cold and dreary winter day, working out at a small health club in Quakertown, when the owner came up to him and asked him if he had ever heard of Spinning. Josh said he had not, but he was interested because he dreaded riding outdoors in winter—not only are the days short and the wind biting, but your feet grow cold and numb and your nose runs in the icy air. Josh thought maybe he could substitute Spinning for at least some of his rides outside. So the owner of the club bought the special Spinning bikes and, as soon as Josh became certified as a Spinning instructor, he taught classes after spending his day training.

Josh was hooked. It was the first time he could remember when he had worked with people other than athletes, but he liked the challenge.

"I said, 'You know what—this is a good program.' I was so used to being around really fit human beings, and it was always *me* being coached. Suddenly, the roles were reversed." He discovered how difficult it can be to encourage people to push themselves. He found that often the people who took his classes either weren't interested in working hard or did not really grasp what he was asking them to do. Most of them just went through the motions. He would look around at his Spinning class and see a few "endorphin junkies." But the others, he remarked, "they just don't want to go there. They just sit on a bike and roll their legs."

He soon discovered the motivational effects of heart-rate monitors, which inspired people to push themselves harder than they thought was possible.

"For me, it was funny. I had been training with some of the best cyclists in the world, but it was Spinning that brought heart-rate monitors to me." Now, more and more professional cyclists, including Lance Armstrong, use the devices. "That's the only way to gauge your training," Josh explains, and the only way to avoid spending time on a bike when you're not putting in enough effort to improve performance—an occupational hazard for bicyclists, who can easily convince themselves they are working harder than they really are. "We call it 'junk miles,' " Josh says.

In 1998, after Josh had been teaching Spinning for about a year, he heard about a charity Spinning ride in Baltimore that was going to be led by Johnny G himself. "A friend of mine was, like, 'Hey, dude, let's check this out,' " Josh says. So the two of them paid their $110 registration fee and drove to Baltimore for the two-hour ride.

"It was different than I expected. I came out of there pretty intrigued," Josh admits. Johnny G, he adds, "is a pretty good motivator. He was out walking the crowd, touching people, working the ride. There was a lot of energy in the room. I was totally digging it."

Johnny noticed Josh and his friend, Jeff Rudder. They were wearing racing jerseys and they had just completed the Altoona Stage Race, the largest stage race in the country, so they were at a peak of fitness, and it showed. Toward the end of the ride, Johnny G announced that the group was going to do five hundred jumps.

"I was, like, 'Okay,' " Josh says. Then Johnny called Josh and Jeff to the front of the room, took his own bike off the stage, and asked the two young men to lead the group. They enthusiastically complied. "I was just whaling through the jumps," Josh tells me.

Two weeks later, Johnny G called the health club where Josh worked and within two months Josh was on a plane to Los Angeles for a special Johnny G camp where he learned to be what is called a "master presenter." Presenters, in the fitness business, are fit and attractive people who train instructors and show up to lead charity rides and special events that encourage health-club owners to institute programs like Spinning. Masters are at the top of the heap.

"The master-presenter thing has been wonderful," Josh says. "It changed my life. As stupid as it sounds, I was like this cocky young athlete. I didn't give a crap about Mrs. Smith coming in the door. But then I started understanding it." He began to realize that he had the power to introduce people to fitness, to change their lives, to remake their bodies. He recalled what the training director told him when he was learning to be a master presenter: "You've got to put in words what you feel on a road bike. What do you get out of training? What is it like?" And that, Josh says, is what let him understand what his goals were. "If I can be around the few people who want to go there, I can help them change their lives."

He wants people to get beyond the tedious treadmill-walking, the moderate exercise, the feeling that exercise is something you have an obligation to do for your health. He worries that few have any idea what it is like to push hard. "There's no education," he says. And so he wants people to experience exercise for what it can be, something that he sees as a transforming experience. I ask him to explain.

"It's just that feeling of fitness. It's the extreme end of life,

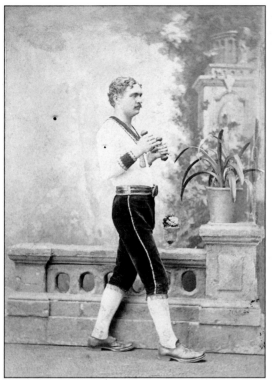

Prof. W. N. Lake, a century pedestrian from 1870, walking with dumbbells.

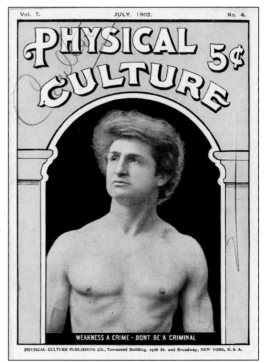

Bernarr Macfadden on the cover of his magazine in July 1902.

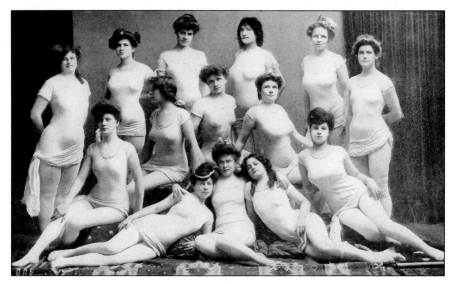

The finalists in Bernarr Macfadden's 1904 contest for the "perfect woman," from the souvenir program, *The Human Form Divine*.

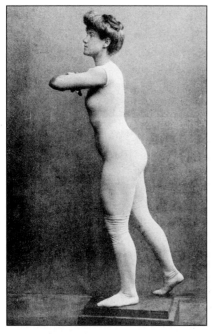

Emma Newkirk, winner of Bernarr Macfadden's contest in 1904 for "the best and most perfectly formed woman." The photo appeared in the contest's souvenir program, *The Human Form Divine*.

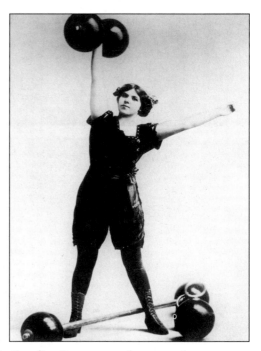

Carolyn Baumann, the most famous student of gym owner and strongman Louis Attila, in about 1915.

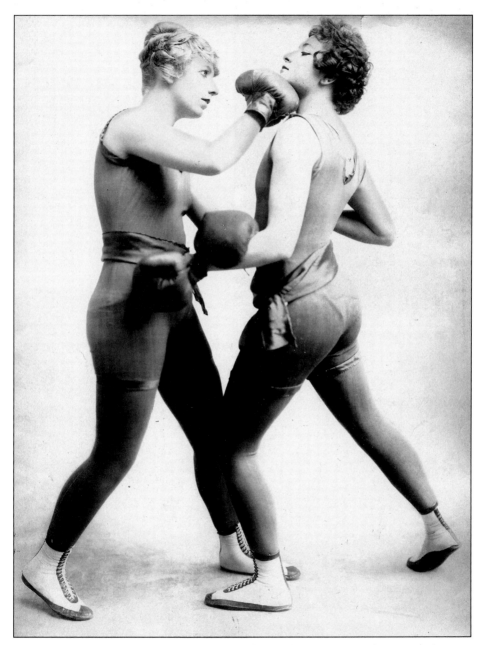

Female boxers Ruth Murphy and Vera Roehm at the Winter Garden, around 1920.

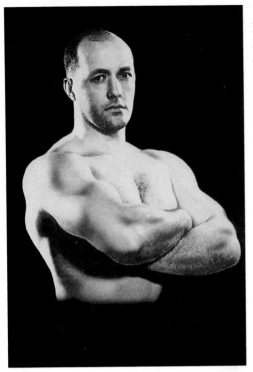

Bob Hoffman, founder of a weight lifting and nutritional supplement empire, in a publicity photo from the late 1930s. The photo was altered to make him look more manly—his muscles were shaded so they appear larger and extra hair was drawn on his head and chest.

Pudgy Stockton, a habitué of Muscle Beach in California, became a body building star in the 1940s. She was on the cover of forty-two magazines, wrote a column on lifting weights, and opened her own gym, for women only.

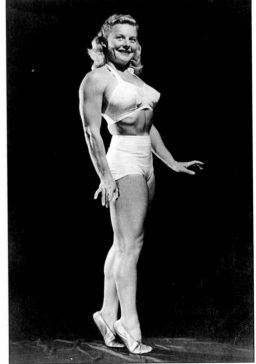

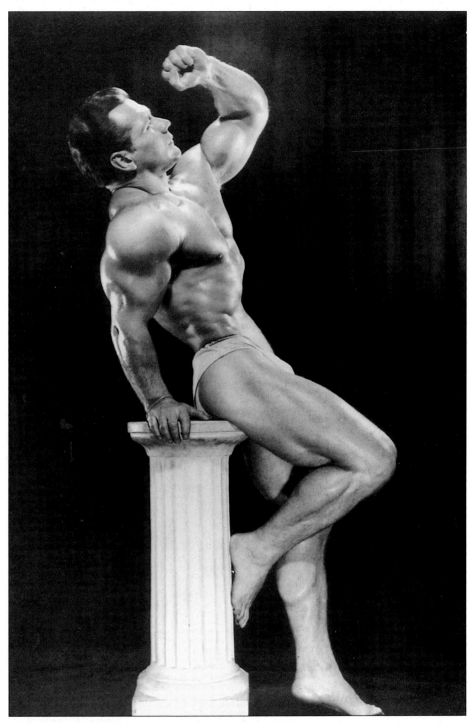

John Grimek, a cult figure for male bodybuilders, in a 1945 photo that Bob Hoffman deemed "the greatest muscle picture ever shown."

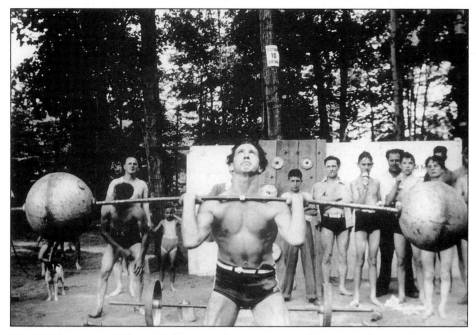

Joe Weider at age eighteen, lifting weights in Montreal.

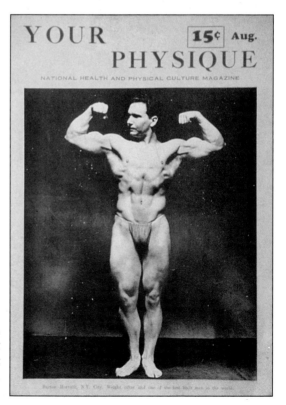

The first issue of *Your Physique*, the magazine Joe Weider launched when he was just seventeen years old.

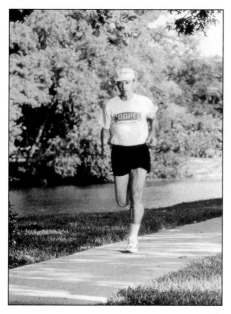

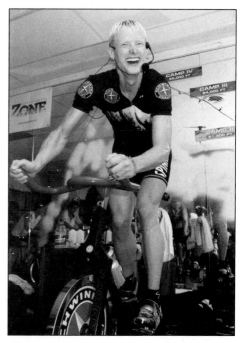

Kenneth Cooper, at age sixty-seven, running along a one-mile trail at his Cooper Aerobics Center in Dallas in 1998.

Josh Taylor leading the Mount Everest ride in April of 2001, chuckling demonically as he urges the participants on.

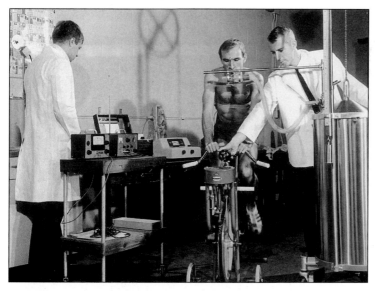

Dave Costill, at age thirty, testing the physiology of college senior Ken Sparks in 1968. Sparks, a world-class 800-meter runner, continued to run after college, setting records in the mile and the 800-meter races when he was forty-seven.

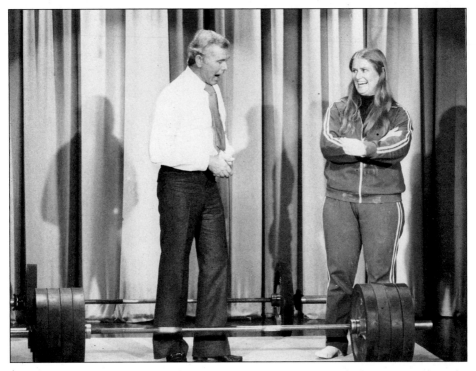

Jan Todd on Johnny Carson's *Tonight* show in 1978. She lifted 415 pounds eight times in a row, but Johnny could not budge the weight without the help of two other men.

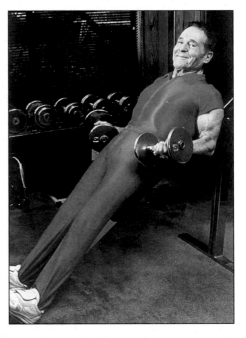

Jack LaLanne, at age eighty-five, in his home gym, where he lifts weights for an hour each morning.

pushing yourself to the very edge, feeling what your body can deal with and what your mind can deal with. You're just absolutely on the rivet. You're just living fully."

One aspect of the Spinning program is the focus on "energy zones," in which classes are asked to keep their heart rates at specific levels. Participants learn endurance one day, as an instructor tells them to sustain a heart rate of 65 to 70 percent of their maximum for most of the class. They would do intervals the next day, moving their heart rate between 65 and 92 percent of its maximum, and strength the next day, with heart rates in the 75 to 85 percent zone. There are also so-called race days, with very high heart rates, 80 to 92 percent of its maximum, when it is as if one is in a race for the entire class. And there are recovery days, calling for a low heart rate between 50 and 65 percent. The rates are a bit low for experienced athletes, Josh admits, explaining that the program is supposed to be for everyone, whatever their fitness level. He has argued with Johnny G's company, Mad Dogg Athletics, that there should be more of a range of rates, to no avail. But for the most part, as Josh soon recognized, those who were used to exercising strenuously worked at higher rates and many who were not used to exercising worked at lower ones, regardless of what the instructor said.

Josh was fascinated. "Spinning gives the everyday person the opportunity to train like a pro," he tells me. But then he began to wonder: What was the point of the energy zones? It was not as if the group was training for an athletic competition. "I got to the point where I was, like, 'Okay. Where am I taking these people?'"

One day, in the summer of 2000, Josh was musing over this question with a friend, Bill Perrault, a solidly built man with short, bleached-blond hair who is also a bicycle racer and runs the Spinning programs at two Pennsylvania gyms. "I remember sitting in a chair and looking out the window and thinking,

'Where could we go?' " Then it popped into his head: Mount
Everest. He could use that mountain, the biggest challenge of
them all, as the symbol and the goal for a ride that would require
serious, focused training. He could bring people into the world of
athletic competition—even if they were only competing against
themselves—to see how hard they could push themselves.

Of course, the ride would always be missing that real element
of competition that drives athletes. But for some, the idea of competition is enough to make them stop before they ever really start.
So maybe this sort of pseudo-competition is the perfect compromise. "It's never going to become an issue of, 'I can't keep up,' "
Josh pointed out. "The only person you're going to be fighting
with is yourself."

Josh had some tough decisions to make about this Mount
Everest event. How long could people ride, pushing themselves at
an athlete's level of effort? And how hard could he really make
them work? What sort of event would require training yet not be
impossible for most people to complete?

He decided that it would be a four-hour Spinning climb, like
riding a bike up a mountain for four hours. "I said, 'Okay, a four-
hour climb. You have to *really* train for that. There is no way that
just killing yourself in Spinning class for forty minutes a day is
going to do it. I am going to take all those people sitting in America someplace else.' "

He began reading obsessively about actual climbs up Mount
Everest, poring over magazine articles and two books, the 1997
best-seller *Into Thin Air: A Personal Account of the Mount Everest Disaster* by Jon Krakauer, and a 1997 National Geographic
book, *Everest: Mountain Without Mercy*. He learned how people
trained to climb Everest, and he learned what it was like to make
that treacherous climb—what the paths climbers had taken were,
where the base camp was, and where other camps where climbers
could rest were. He learned where the air got so thin that almost
everyone needed oxygen, and where the mountain was so high
that it was above the clouds.

"This was a test of yourself," Josh says. "It's giving the every-day person something to aim for. Even an athlete—even me. I've raced up some pretty big hills but I've never been up a four-hour climb, that's for sure." He immediately thought of Sharon and Evolutions as a place to hold the event. He had met Sharon LaForge through Spinning, and had even taught some classes at Evolutions Fitness. And Sharon, as Josh predicted, was ready to go. Soon, she, Josh, and Bill Perrault were mapping it out, offer-ing a special training program to those who wanted to try this ultimate challenge.

Josh did not ask people to provide assurances from their doc-tor that they could safely train. After all, he said, people in Spin-ning classes work at their own level—that's the point of Spinning.

"The whole point of the Everest ride was to give someone an opportunity to climb their own hill," Josh says. "You don't have to be an athlete to enter."

seven

MOUNT EVEREST

The training schedule that Josh and Bill Perrault devised—the one Bill and I avidly followed—lasted for eleven weeks. They planned it so that we would accustom our bodies to increasingly longer rides with increasingly higher resistance on the pedals, training as though we were actually climbing longer and steeper hills outdoors. They wanted us to be as strong as possible, so in addition to the Spinning training, we were supposed to lift weights at least twice a week. One day was to emphasize the lower body and abdominals, and the other day the upper body and abdominals.

As a guide, they gave us a few sheets with diagrams of weight-lifting routines. I followed what I was already doing, which was more demanding than what they were suggesting. For example, I do squats, hoisting a weight-loaded barbell across my shoulders and squatting, my rear end thrust out. That works the muscles of the thighs—the quadriceps and hamstrings. It also works the hip flexors and gluteals. I do bench presses, lying faceup on a bench and grasping a weighted barbell that I lower to my chest and lift up again. That works the chest muscles. Or I'll do push-ups. There are dozens of ways to work each muscle and I often vary what I do, depending on whether my favorite equipment is in use or whether one or another exercise appeals to me that day. The only constant is that I do three different exercises for each muscle group, like the chest muscles. I repeat each exercise ten to twelve times, then rest briefly, do it again, rest again, and then do a third set. It is time-consuming—I often spend about three hours a week lifting weights—but I like, even crave, the effort. To train for the actual Spinning ride, we were to take two to three Spinning classes during the week, and on the weekends there were special training rides. They started out at two hours, increasing to two and a half hours. They peaked with a three-hour ride, then decreased to two and a half hours. They were held on Friday nights and on Saturday and Sunday afternoons—you had to choose one and sign up in advance to hold a place.

While we rode, we were supposed to experiment with foods and sports drinks to see what we liked best. Bill and I discovered tubes of sports gels, which are super-sweet, like eating the icing from a cake. I like icing, but these gels were over the top when we tried them at home, a bit too intense to be appealing even to me. Yet when we ate them while we were exercising, they were great—their flavor seemed perfect, and since we feared that a long ride could use so much energy that we would have to supply our bodies with carbohydrates, the gels promised to be useful. At least you do not have to chew them while you're breathing hard.

I was curious about the three-hour training ride because I remembered so vividly how wretched we had felt after the three-hour charity ride. This ride seemed a lot harder. It was to include one hour of endurance riding at 60 to 80 percent of our maximum heart rate, an hour's worth of long climbs, each lasting 15 to 25 minutes at 80 to 90 percent of our maximum heart rate, and then another hour of endurance riding. I had found in Spinning classes that I could get my heart rate up to 80 to 90 percent of my maximum; but to maintain it for long periods with hill climbs—a fairly slow pedal speed with high resistance—seemed painful even to contemplate and impossibly hard to do.

Bill and I arrived at Evolutions on a Saturday morning. The ride was to go from eleven a.m. till two p.m., led by Kathryn's friend Bill Fox. He came from Middletown, New York, a two-hour drive away, but he was accustomed to showing up in New

Jersey on weekends, when he would embark on day-long rides with Kathryn and her group. By day, he was a technician in a physics lab at IBM, but the rest of the time he was a serious bicyclist who rode "double centuries"—200 miles in a single day's ride. (Bill died in June of 2002, while training for a 200-mile ride, a double century, crashing his bike while riding downhill alone. Though he was wearing a helmet, he suffered fatal head injuries. My husband Bill and I, along with hundreds of others who knew Bill Fox, however briefly, were heartbroken. It was a sobering reminder of the dangers of road bicycling, where a flat tire or a pothole in the road can send you flying over your handlebars as you speed down a steep hill.)

For the Mount Everest ride, Bill Fox was in his element. He had come to Spinning because he hated riding outdoors in winter and Spinning seemed to offer a way of staying in shape during the coldest months. He hoped that a hard Spinning class could give him the euphoric feeling he craved from vigorous exercise. But he was dismayed to find that the instructors at his gym were former aerobics instructors who had never ridden bikes and who had no idea how to sit on a bike and how to move. So, he decided, if he wanted a Spinning class for serious bicyclists, he'd have to teach it himself.

Bill Fox was middle-aged and balding, wore glasses, and had an amazing ability to sweat. His taste in music ran to jazz and Janis Joplin—he remarked once that if someone had told him when he was young that he would be Spinning to Janis Joplin, he would have shot himself. All the while, throughout the three-hour ride, he sweated, and sweated. Sweat dripped off his nose, off his chin, falling in a steady rain to form vast puddles on the floor. He wore a microphone and headset so we could hear him over the music, but he sweated so much that Sharon had to keep replacing the foam rubber over the microphone's mouthpiece.

What amazed me was that my husband and I not only enjoyed the three-hour ride but we felt wonderful afterward. Training seemed to be working.

I had lots of questions, of course. Why, for example, did we have to eat? If I can go five, six, sometimes seven hours between lunch and dinner on an ordinary day and feel perfectly fine, why should it be necessary to eat during a two- or three-hour Spinning ride? And what sort of food was best? Why do we need to replace fluids while we ride, and why is it so hard to ride when the room is warm?

Everyone at Evolutions seems to have a different idea of how much and when to eat and drink during the training rides. Kathryn favors Cytomax, a powder you mix with water to replace electrolytes and fluids. Others tote large bottles of Gatorade. Some like bagels and bananas. Others like energy bars, like Zone Bars and Power Bars or Cliff Bars. Bill and I stay with our gels, deciding we like a brand called Gu, experimenting mostly with different flavors.

I can't shake the feeling that all of this is a bit ridiculous, that we are only pseudo-athletes pretending to train. Mount Everest is not a race, after all, and we will only be competing against ourselves. It seemed to me that maybe all this experimenting with different foods and drinks is a type of game-playing. Maybe, just as we are pretending to be in an athletic contest, we also are pretending to be eating like champions. It seemed possible that despite the food and drink obsessions so many of us have, it makes no difference what we eat or drink, or even *if* we eat or drink during the ride.

Exercise physiologists have spent decades trying to answer the kinds of questions I'm asking. So perhaps, I think, they might have some scientific data to resolve them. And maybe the thing to do is to watch an exercise physiologist in action, someone who has a reputation among other scientists for trying to do the research correctly. When I ask researchers who they would recommend, one name keeps coming up: Dave Costill. I knew about him, of course, and I had already phoned him several times to inquire about exercise physiology. But I had never met him and had never set foot in a human-performance lab. So, Dave Costill it would be. The coauthor of a leading textbook on exercise physiology, the author of more than four hundred papers, the recipient of awards from groups ranging from the American College of Sports Medicine, of which he had been president, to the magazine *Runner's World*, he seemed the natural person to turn to for reliable data.

Costill, says Paul Ribisl, the chairman of health and exercise science at Wake Forest University, "is just a superb person as well as one of the top exercise physiologists." Ribisl adds: "He's certainly done some of the most interesting work and had a powerful influence on the field." Costill's specialty, Ribisl explains, is to apply the methods of science to a field that, sadly, had often neglected them. "He's basically allowed the science to dispel the misconceptions."

I visit him at his lab at Ball State University, in the tiny Indiana town of Muncie, about a two-hour drive through farmlands from the Dayton airport. It is a town of frame houses and a deserted business district, a town dominated by the red brick buildings of the university. There, in one of the newer buildings, right next to an indoor swimming pool, is the two-story structure that houses the Human Performance Laboratory where Costill and his colleagues do their work.

It is a quintessentially masculine domain, peopled by strapping young graduate students who love science but are also serious athletes, drawn to the field by their own questions about how to improve performance, a question that often stems from their own attempts to train for competition. In their spare time they swim competitively, or ride bikes, or do rock climbing.

I arrive at what proves to be a particularly inopportune moment. An important donor to the perennially cash-strapped program has just shown up and wants to talk about the status of the research. A reporter, of course, can wait. At any other school, someone would ask if I'd like a cup of coffee, or would I like to go to the library, or sit in an office somewhere and read some reprints of recent research papers. But this is the Human Performance Laboratory, and people here have different ideas about how to treat a guest. Would I care to swim? Lift weights? Run?

How perfect. It is a crisp, clear day and I'd already spent hours in airports and sitting in a cramped seat on a small plane and then driving a rental car. Without hesitation, I tell Costill I'd like to run. I go to my car to get my running clothes—I always carry workout clothes with me. I change in a ladies' room in the building, which turns out to be equipped with lockers and a shower. Before I leave, some of those extremely fit-looking graduate students ask me how far I want to go, then direct me to an appropriate path along the river just beyond the campus.

I return forty-five minutes later, shower, and, still with that sense of exercise-induced exhilaration, sit down to my interview with Costill.

He is an unlikely person to be a leader in science in these days when the scientific stars are molecular biologists and genome decoders and stem-cell experts from biotechnology firms and leading universities. A modest Midwesterner, he is the son of a machinist. Costill started out as a high school teacher and a coach, and only later went back to school to get a Ph.D. in exercise physiology. It is a world unto itself, a place where prominent researchers find themselves in schools that are almost backwaters in the world of high-tech science. Its practitioners borrow methods from the more sophisticated areas of science, but their work is largely unknown to the rest of the scientific world. Most of the research is carried out by people for whom exercise is an avocation as well as a vocation. It is a small world, and Costill stands out as one of its grand old men.

Costill is a swimmer, tall and lean. He works out in the pool each day at lunch and swims in masters' meets. His swimming times are as fast now as they were when he was in college more than forty years ago. (He attributes this to better training, not to a miraculous ability to stave off the effects of aging.)

Questions about his own training and innate athletic abilities drew Costill to the field of exercise science. Why, he asked, was he not a better runner? He tried training with expert marathon runners, matching them mile for mile. But when the race day came, they left him far behind. So, he began asking, why are some people so much better at certain sports than others? Is there an inborn physiological difference between, say, a sprinter and a marathon runner? How should people train to maximize their performance? Why does the body adapt with training?

"I wanted to find out why I was such a bad runner," Costill told me. "The best I ever did in a marathon was 3 hours and 15 minutes. I was training seventy miles a week, but I just couldn't get any better. I wanted to know what made those other guys so good."

That was at the start of his long career. He investigated, among other things, the two types of muscle fibers, so-called fast-twitch and slow-twitch. Fast-twitch muscles contract quickly when they are stimulated by nerves. They are used for speed. Slow-twitch muscles contract more slowly but have a larger energy supply so they can continue contracting longer. They are used for endurance.

Most people have about equal numbers of muscle type. But the gifted endurance athletes, like champion marathon runners, appear to have a predominance of slow-twitch fibers and the best sprinters seem to have mostly fast-twitch fibers. Costill, and everyone else in his lab, tested their own muscles repeatedly, driving a small borelike device into a muscle like the quadriceps in the front of the leg, pulling out a small plug of muscle, putting the tissue on a microscope slide, and poring over it. Costill quickly learned why he never got very good at distance running. He has the muscles of a sprinter, mostly fast-twitch ones.

The muscle-fiber distinction, I tell him, could be pretty important to young people first starting out in a sport. Why set yourself up for failure by going into an endurance sport, when you are built for sprinting, or vice versa? Does he ever test people and tell them what their muscle fibers look like? No, he says, except as part of research studies. Every now and then, parents will wander into the lab or write to him and ask him to test their child, but he explains that he does research, he is not selling a diagnostic service. To Costill, what matters is the science, not its application as yet another product to be sold to athletes and would-be athletes.

As the years went by, Costill never veered from his mission to understand the science of exercise physiology and human performance. He was my sort of scientist, emphasizing how to improve performance. Central to his research, and his own personal interests in athletic performance, were questions regarding the physiological effects of training. Like everyone else in this field, his studies were done on a shoestring, with budgets that are almost ludicrously small by the standards of scientific research. As a consequence, Costill and others who asked the same sorts of questions, were forced to do small studies; their experiments involved only a handful of subjects, with a dozen or fewer young men in a typical study. Yet time after time, in numerous variations on the same experiment, the answers came out the same. And they made biological sense. So the data, although less than ideal, add up to a consistent and credible story of how and why certain aspects of training really can change one's body and improve performance.

One question that Costill and others asked is, Why do muscles get tired? Are they running out of fuel, and if so, could they be refreshed if provided with more fuel during exercise?

Theory told Costill that endurance athletes—and I guess my Mount Everest training might put me in that category—run the risk of depleting their muscles of glycogen, their primary energy source, as they call on their muscles to perform hour after hour. Some athletes try to store extra glycogen by eating huge amounts of carbohydrates, which the body metabolizes into sugar, before an event. And this works, to an extent, but there is only so much that the body can store.

Costill noticed that during a long-distance running or cycling event, blood glucose levels can start to drop, and that, he thought, might contribute to fatigue. He started doing experiments with bicyclists and runners, documenting repeatedly the fact that sugar can boost an endurance athlete's performance.

In one study, published in 1980 in the *International Journal of Sports Medicine*, he compared how well a group of bicyclists fared during a two-hour ride when they were given carbohydrates, in this case a sweet sports drink, with the performance of a group that drank artificially sweetened flavored water. Every fifteen minutes, the athletes sipped their drinks. For the first ninety minutes, it made no difference what they drank. Both groups of athletes weakened gradually, their power output diminished by about 10 percent. Then, the bicyclists who were getting real sugar in their drinks started getting stronger, ending the ride with a greater power output than they had at the beginning. But those who had the placebo continued to tire, dropping nearly another 10 percent in their power output.

In another study, published in 1988 in *Medical and Scientific Aspects of Cycling. Proceedings of 1986 World Congress*, Costill asked young men to ride bikes for four hours. He gave them a sugar solution before they began and after one, two, and three hours of riding. He asked the ten young men in the study to ride again, this time giving them artificially sweetened water, although the test subjects themselves didn't know which ride was the one with real sugar for fuel and which one was not. At the end of each ride, the men were asked to sprint, pedaling as fast as they could, at maximum effort, until they could go no faster.

Those given the sugared drinks used less glycogen from their vastus lateralis muscle, a part of the quadriceps muscle, located on the outer part of the thigh, which extends the leg during running—and pedaling a bike. They also were able to sprint for nearly twice as long—going for about forty seconds—than they could when they had only artificially sweetened water to drink. Costill cautions, however, that these results do not mean that sugar can improve performance when the muscles already have plenty of glycogen stored in them; only that extra sugar can overcome glycogen depletion.

So the sports gels we were swallowing probably helped us. What about water, I asked. I remembered Ted Corbitt's story, how he accidentally discovered that he was so dehydrated, able to keep running only when he stuck out his tongue to catch falling snow.

We were hardly doing the equivalent of Corbitt's thirty-mile run. We had water bottles during those long training rides, and Sharon was constantly roaming the room, refilling them. Yet, I wondered, how much water did we really need, and why? When Costill first began his long career in exercise physiology, water was considered an illegal performance-enhancer for marathon runners. The marathon rules said that no one could drink water for the first 10 kilometers (6.2 miles) of a race, and after that the runners had to stash their water along the route, or carry it with them. There were no water stations.

It was 1968, and Costill, newly arrived at Ball State, had a student who was an alternate on the U.S. Olympic marathon team. Marathons were less popular then and few athletes attempted them. "There were only two hundred people in the U.S. who could run a marathon and he knew all of them," Costill says, and in that he saw an opportunity. "I decided I wanted to do a research project looking at dehydration and overheating," he says. With the assistance of his student, he went to the Olympic training camp to study the elite runners.

In those days, marathons were held in the summer and, not surprisingly, runners suffered from heat stroke. "They were totally collapsing," he says. Costill took their rectal temperatures before and after the race and discovered that their body temperatures were soaring to 103, 104, 105, and, in one astonishing case, 109 degrees. That man, miraculously, survived the experience, although his temperature was truly high enough to kill him.

Costill looked to see what they were drinking, and it turned out to be almost nothing. People would lose twelve pounds or more, a gallon of fluid, all because of the marathon rule. "It was a stupid rule," Costill remarks, and after he documented, and others confirmed, its dangerous effects, it was changed so runners could get as much water as they wanted at regularly spaced water stations. In 1968, some races were allowing fluids, but not the Olympic trials, Costill says. But by 1972, he adds, the no-fluid rule had been abandoned internationally.

You lose water by sweating. The more water that is lost, the worse one's performance. That is because your blood volume goes down when fluids are depleted, which decreases blood pressure. But if blood pressure goes down, physiologists say, less blood can get to the muscles, and so they get less glucose and oxygen and less blood gets to the surface of the skin for cooling. You try to compensate—your heart beats faster. But since less blood is getting to your skin, your body is getting hotter and hotter. You are forced to slow down.

That explains why I feel so much better if I can put my Spinning bike near a fan. The fan dries the sweat from my skin, cooling my blood and helping me avoid part of this vicious cycle. I've never understood the people who sweat but stay away from fans in gyms, afraid of getting a chill. Now I feel justified. It seems that a chill is exactly what you should want.

I remember fruitless arguments over fans in gyms. I used to go to Manhattan Plaza Health Club, a gym in New York that had rotating fans over its StairMaster machines. The protocol was that if you wanted a fan and no one around you objected, you could pull a chain and turn the fan on. But almost everyone objected, afraid they would get a chill. Some people would drape towels around their necks to ward off what they thought were dangerous breezes.

At my Gold's Gym in New Jersey, one trainer used to insist it was unhealthy to have a fan blow air on you as you exercised, and she would turn off the fan when she was on the floor. It never made sense to me—you are sweating to try to get your body temperature down. A fan will speed cooling so you can sweat less, lose less fluid, and, I thought, feel better. I used to ask her to at least let the clients decide if they wanted a fan to blow on them. But every time, there would be one person, at least, who said "no fan," and off it would stay.

Even worse, of course, is exercising when the air is hot. Randy Vey, the owner of the Gold's where I am a member, told me that clients complained if he kept the room chilly. I suggested that it was easier for members who were cold to wear sweatshirts and stay warm than it was for those of us who were hot from working out to cool down. Once again, I find, research vindicates me, but gyms are a business and if most clients want no fans and warm rooms, that's what they will get.

Surprisingly, you can actually overcome the effects of a warm room by drinking—and sweating, profusely. In one experiment, athletes tried to run for six hours on a treadmill in a room kept at 104 degrees. Those who were deprived of fluids could not do it. Within five hours, they had to stop—their heart rates were sky high and they were completely exhausted. Others, who were drinking water all the while, kept up their effort for the entire time, and their heart rates hardly rose as the hours wore on.

But you cannot count on your thirst to tell you how much to drink. Thirst, it turns out, kicks in after dehydration is under way, and it may take twenty-four to forty-eight hours to drink enough fluids to make up for the losses.

Some extreme examples of the problem of drinking enough fluids were related at a 1977 conference at Ball State. C. H. Wyndham of Marshalltown, Transvaal, South Africa, reported the experience of one of his country's best runners in a marathon in Athens in the early 1970s. The day was hot and humid, but his coach had forgotten to take along anything for the runner to drink during the race. "As a result, the runner ran the entire race

without any fluids. He ran to twenty miles, where he became totally disoriented."

Alan Claremont, a runner and teacher at the University of
Wisconsin in Madison, told of a nationally ranked runner who
could run a marathon in 2 hours and 15 minutes. But he had
problems with fainting when he ran marathons on hot days. So
they asked him to run in the lab. After 1 hour 22 minutes, running at a 6-minute-mile pace, he had sweated so much that his
body weight, already low at 104 pounds, was reduced by 5 percent. Claremont noted that if the man had continued to run for
another hour, he would have lost 7 percent of his body weight
from sweating and would have been so dehydrated that he might
well have fainted. "Thus," Claremont concluded, "it should be
emphasized that frequent fluid feedings beyond satiation are essential for maximum endurance performance."

Now I know. We have to stay cool on the Mount Everest ride,
and we have to eat—the sports gels seem ideal, and it is hard to
drink too much water. We may be playing at being athletes, but
we still need to take care to eat and drink enough if we want to
finish the ride feeling good.

So we follow Josh's training schedule. We follow the advice to
rest for several days before the Mount Everest ride, and to eat a
diet that is loaded with carbohydrates. We eat pasta for dinner,
but that is our usual dinner on weeknights anyway because we
can prepare it so quickly. As for training diets and counting
grams of protein and carbohydrates and fat for weeks on end,
that was not suggested, and we felt no need to complicate our
training unnecessarily. This was a ride to see if we could meet our
own personal challenge; we were not out to shave seconds off a
race time and beat a competitor. Even if we were, I am not convinced that a meticulous diet would make a difference. I put my
faith in weight lifting and, most important, in those training rides.

On the big day, April 21, 2001, Bill and I arrive early at Evolutions Fitness. We wanted to be sure we could grab bikes in front of a fan. This time, we knew there would be a crowd in the large cement-floored room—for the first time, all forty of us who had been training would be together—and we were worried that the place would get hot. To accommodate us, Sharon had rented twenty extra bikes from another gym, supplementing the twenty she owned.

The forty bikes are arranged in concentric circles around a platform in front of one of the walls. That is where Josh and Bill Perrault will perch on their bikes, leading us on the ride. Bill and I choose bikes on the far right as you face the platform, with Bill's bike in front of mine. A large fan is directly behind us.

Bill and I are dressed for comfort. We wear our skintight black bicycling shorts to prevent chafing, and matching fluorescent-green sleeveless bicycling jerseys. The jerseys have zippers down the front so we can open them as we get hot. They are made of sweat-wicking netted fabric, and, best of all, they have a long pocket across the back where we can tuck our tubes of sugary sports gel.

Sharon, Kathryn, and Sue pass out Breathe Right nasal strips, those bands of plastic encased in an adhesive pad that you can put over your nose to open up your airways. We could slip them over our noses, they said, for a more complete Mount Everest experience, allowing us to simulate oxygen deprivation when we had gotten to a place on the mountain where climbers would be gasping for air.

As the time comes to start the ride, when all of us are seated and ready to go, the buzz of excited conversation is replaced by a palpable silence and we really are transported into another world. The bare-bones Spinning room is transformed; it reminds me of a high school gym decorated for a big dance. The plate-glass windows are covered with translucent paper, dimming the bright daylight and blocking our view of the asphalt parking lot outside. The walls are draped with Tibetan prayer flags colored blue, yellow, and green. Sharon has set up a screen in front of the room and is playing a video of a real Mount Everest climb. The sound is turned off so what we get are images of the cold, snowy, and forbidding mountain and climbers in their bulky clothes laboriously trudging up its slopes. Behind the low platform, where Josh Taylor and Bill Perrault are sitting on their Spinning bikes, is an outline of Mount Everest, traced in blue Christmas lights, with the base camp and four rest camps marked with little colored flags—white, green, yellow, red, and rainbow colored. The base camp, where we start, is at 17,600 feet. As we climb, we pass over the Khumbu icefall to reach the first rest camp, at 19,500 feet. Rest camp two is at 21,300 feet, camp three is at 24,000 feet, and camp four is at 26,000 feet. From there the climb takes a sharp jog upward, with a frighteningly steep path to the top, at 29,028 feet.

Candles are burning, Eastern music is playing. I later learn that Josh spent forty hours choosing the music, Eastern and techno, for the ride and putting it together to lead us through the four-hour climb.

The ride begins, with an all too short warm-up on the bikes before we start. Josh tells us to sit back on the bike seat, to turn up the resistance, and get our heart rates up to 80 percent of their maximums. We are climbing. Before long, it becomes unbearable, my quadriceps muscles at the front of my thighs are tiring and my hamstrings at the back of my thighs feel like they can pull no longer. Then Bill Perrault tells us to stand, to climb leaning over the bike, our backs flat, pushing down on the pedals. At last, relief. When you stand, it is easier to push the pedals because you can take full advantage of your body weight to bear down at each pedal stroke. Too soon, he tells us to sit again. We push on the pedals, pulling up on the backstroke, listening to the music, listening to Josh and Bill's patter about what goes on in a real Everest climb and, all the while, concentrating on keeping our heart rates up, pedaling at a constant rate, keeping our form, maintaining our effort.

We climb to simulate the path of the mountain, and I watch its outline, knowing that sooner or later we have to get to that first rest camp. When it comes, when Josh and Bill announce that we are there, we have a five-minute period of blessed relief. Pedaling with a light resistance, never leaving my bike, I rip open a tube of gel, sucking it into my mouth. I pull open the nozzle of my water bottle, open my mouth wide, and squirt water down my throat. Meanwhile, Sharon, Kathryn, and Sue walk among us, offering water, sports drinks, sports bars, fresh fruit, and bagels.

All too soon, the rest is over and we are off again. Grinning devilishly, Josh tells us to increase the resistance on our pedals and to resume the climb. Bill Perrault takes over, issuing instructions. Stand up, he says, lean forward over the handlebars. It feels so good to get up from the seat. Now, he says, increase the resistance. We do. Now, he tells us, sit down again and don't touch the resistance knob. It is agonizing; the resistance is higher than before, when I thought I could hardly go on. Somehow, we prevail. Then he instructs us to stand again. Relief—I can do this, I tell myself. Now, he says, turn that resistance knob again. I turn it. We pedal along for a few minutes. Sit down, Bill says, and don't touch the resistance.

Over and over we repeat this excruciating move. Each time I think, "I can't," but each time, somehow, I do it. Meanwhile, Sharon and Kathryn and Sue wander through the room, refilling water bottles, offering food. Bill and I take only water—we have our gels tucked in our back pockets and every forty-five minutes we open another and suck it down. When we get above the clouds on our simulated climb, Sharon, Kathryn, and Sue emerge, dumping dry ice in buckets of water to create a mist. It lingers in the air, ethereal, making it easier than ever to be transported out of East Brunswick, New Jersey, and into a world where all that matters is to keep pushing the pedals, watching my heart rate, letting the music help take me into the athlete's world. I am unaware of the others in the room; all that matters is this intense effort and this determination not to let up.

The hours pass, a haze of effort and more effort. I know Bill is in front of me. I know Bill Fox is sitting in the middle of the room, next to Laura, who is one of the regulars in Arline's Saturday classes. I know that Anna Hess, the Spinning instructor from Gold's, is directly across the room from me. And Arnold Cantor, an amiable man who hates the fans, is somewhere at the very back of the room. Yet I have no awareness of them. I have no idea if they are still riding, or if they look tired. All I know is my own pedal strokes, my own heart rate, my own effort. I keep telling myself what Donald Kirkendall had said: "Most people have no idea how hard they can work."

Somehow, the ride is almost at an end. We have passed the fourth rest camp and we are heading straight uphill. We have an hour to go and it is getting harder and harder to keep pedaling. Finally, we are just about there. Ten minutes are left in the four-hour ride. I look at the outline of Everest and see that it takes a sharp turn upward, a vertical climb, almost straight up into thin air. And, yes, Josh tells us, we have arrived at the steepest part of the mountain. He tells us what we have to do—crank up the re-sistance some more and push like we have never pushed before. Each revolution of the pedals should take all the strength we can muster. My pedal resistance is already high and I can hardly imagine turning the knob any more. It will be like pedaling in slow motion. My heart is beating at 85 percent of its maximum rate. I have been going for almost four hours. How much more can I do? Of course, our leaders tell us, it's our climb. "Maybe you won't summit, but that's okay," they say.

Suddenly, the ride is over. Not only did Bill and I get through it, but we feel great. Exhausted, but not drained, more like pleas-antly tired. We climb off our bikes and Josh and Bill lead us in long, languorous stretches to the sounds of New Age music. We put one leg on the seat and lean over it, savoring the delicious hamstring stretch. We do it again, stretching the other hamstring. We stand on one leg, pulling the foot of our other leg to our but-

tocks, stretching our quadriceps. We stand behind the bike, putting one foot against the frame and leaning forward—a stretch
for the calves. Never did it feel so good to stretch muscles.

Finally, we wipe our bikes with a disinfectant spray. I go to the
locker room and peel off my sweat-soaked clothes, changing into
clean and dry sweatpants and a sweatshirt.

We linger for about half an hour, joining the others to eat
some sweet fresh mango slices and chewy bagels, and then we
drive home. Neither Bill nor I feel anything like the bone-tired exhaustion that had dogged us the day we did the three-hour charity ride, yet Mount Everest was a much more challenging event.
We feel good—fatigued, but not depleted. Miraculously, the training had worked. Josh had brought us a little way into his world.
Or so it seemed to us.

My son Stefan, a competitive runner, has a different view.
What we experienced was not the thrill of competition, he tells
us, but the satisfaction of strenuous exertion. And what motivated us was not what motivates athletes. They want to win. He
tells me about one of his coaches who said he knew he could run
a marathon in a respectable time, but he did not just want to be
one of a pack who finishes. He would only race to win. Our
training, Stefan says, was less for a competition than for "a hard
practice."

I write about Mount Everest for the *New York Times*. Soon a
group of executives in Washington call Josh and end up paying
him to lead a private Mount Everest just for them. He does another Mount Everest at a Johnny G Spinning conference in Miami
in January of 2002. Some of the participants, he says, were not at
all fit. When the ride was over, they wept, overwhelmed by what
they had accomplished.

Then I get an e-mail from Richard Friedman, a psychopharmacologist at Cornell Medical School. Did I get a runner's high,
he asks? Well, no, I tell him, I did not. I seem to get a feeling of

almost ecstatic exhilaration—is that a runner's high?—when I exercise at a very high heart rate for more than half an hour. But a
long endurance event, even at 80 to 85 percent of my maximum
effort, does not seem to elicit that feeling. I start to wonder: Does
exercise affect your mind? Does it, as is often claimed, alleviate
depression? Is there such a thing as a runner's high? And, if so,
what causes it? Is it caused by endorphins, as most people say, or
is that yet another exercise myth?

eight

IS THERE A RUNNER'S HIGH?

The folklore has it that vigorous exercise is like a drug. It is supposed to flood the brain with morphine-like chemicals, endorphins, that elicit feelings of euphoria, giving you a so-called runner's high. And this feeling is so fabulous, the fabled theory goes, that those who experience it want to go back for more, and to spread the news of their wonderful discovery. They are supposed to be like drug addicts, hooked on exercise and, in some cases, unable to stop talking about it.

The notion is so widely accepted, it seems, and the endorphin rush so loosely defined, that it is not clear what experience is being described, nor whether the endorphins come from strenuous exercise or just any exercise experience.

The word has even become a verb. Bill Fox, the late Spinning instructor from Middletown, New York, said to me one day in May of 2002 that he had just come back from a fabulous Spinning class with Josh Taylor feeling "endorphinized." No more explanation was necessary. From magazines and newspapers to reference books, the endorphin hypothesis is everywhere.

I glance at a popular bodybuilding magazine, *Men's Fitness*, skimming the usual array of articles on how to lose weight and how to get large, well-defined muscles. There, in a piece titled "Fat-Loss Handbook," I spot it. Adam Drewnowski, director of the nutrition sciences program at the University of Washington, is offering advice on how to resist food cravings. One of his tips is to exercise. "Exercise releases endorphins that can satisfy your physical cravings," he tells the magazine, but the reader is given no additional information—for example, what kind of exercise, or for how long, or at what intensity. And no mention of how anyone knows that it satisfies food cravings. Maybe the word "endorphins" is enough.

My own newspaper, the *New York Times*, cites the endorphin idea repeatedly, sometimes in articles written by medical authorities. In one, Sherwin B. Nuland, a surgeon in New Haven who wrote a best-selling book, *How We Die*, described what happened when, at age sixty-two, he began working out at a gym. He worked with a trainer, lifting weights and running on a treadmill. He says his body looks much better as a result. "And I feel wonderful," he writes. "What is more, I come home from the gym pumped up with endorphins and put in a few hours of very efficient work."

I look up "endorphins" at encyclopedia.com, Columbia University's online encyclopedia. Endorphins, it says, transmit signals in the brain and "have pain-relieving properties similar to morphine." In addition to "behaving as a pain regulator, endorphins are also thought to be connected to physiological processes including euphoric feelings, appetite modulation, and the release of sex hormones. Prolonged, continuous exercise contributes to an increase in production and release of endorphins, resulting in a sense of euphoria that has been popularly labeled 'runner's high.' "

I check to see what the Chemical Heritage Foundation says about endorphins. The group, headquartered in Philadelphia, seeks to educate the public about chemistry and its uses. Among other activities, it produces materials for teachers. Endorphins are part of its module written for middle school and high school students. "Endorphins are thought to be involved in helping your brain experience pleasure. So eating chocolate is thought to make your body produce endorphins. If you decide to burn off that chocolate with some good hard exercise, that will make your body produce endorphins, too. This is why long-distance runners experience 'runner's high.' The harder you exercise, the more endorphins your body makes. No wonder the Odyssey Adventure Racing calls its annual two-day, 100-mile running, hiking, climbing, paddling, and biking race through the mountains of West Virginia the Endorphin Fix."

Cornell University's nutrition division provides a question-and-answer service, Nutriquest, that has been operating since 1991, answering questions that the public poses, although it stopped taking new questions in July 2002. On its Web site, it, too, addresses endorphins and the runner's high: "It has been suggested (and a growing body of scientific evidence would support) that people who are compulsive exercisers become 'addicted' to the endorphins released in their brain during exercise. Endorphins are the natural morphine-like substances produced in the brain on exercising, which make you feel good and decrease your ability to feel pain. Endorphins may also contribute to better muscle function with training.

"Endorphins are thought to be responsible for 'runner's high,' the good feelings a person may experience after running a long distance to near exhaustion. When compulsive exercisers are not exercising, they may experience the discomforts and irritability of endorphin withdrawal, a mild form of morphine withdrawal, as well as the irritability caused by psychological feelings of guilt at not exercising."

Yet even in this limited sample, three expert sources differ in what it takes to achieve a runner's high, although all agree that endorphins are involved. Either you have to exercise for a long time, or you have to do very strenuous exercise, or you have to exercise nearly to exhaustion. Other sources have other variants on ways to achieve a runner's high, many of them so vague about what is required that it is impossible to pin them down.

Then again, there are some amazing stories about addicted runners, related by William P. Morgan, an exercise physiologist at the University of Wisconsin in Madison. He writes that it takes a while for running to become addictive—initially, like smoking, it is unpleasant. "At first, the tobacco and smoke do not taste good, and there may be dizziness and nausea. However, as the smoker progresses from five cigarettes a day to 10, 15, or 20, the stimulus is perceived as pleasurable and the smoker is addicted. In the early days and weeks of a jogging program, individuals may experience many sensations such as dyspnea, muscle soreness, and numerous aches and pains." But those who persist, he says, may find themselves hooked, and sometimes acting as self-destructively as any drug addict.

He provides some, admittedly extreme, case studies. One thirty-five-year-old professor could not take a break from his daily runs, even though he was injured and in extreme pain. Soon, it got so bad that he had to walk downstairs backwards in the morning. "I knew something was wrong, but I just could not give it up—it felt so good," he said. "Finally, I awoke one morning and was unable to even go downstairs backwards." He ended up in surgery for a ruptured Achilles tendon.

A forty-five-year-old man would leave his office at 11:45 a.m. for his daily run, "regardless of what he had on his desk," Morgan relates. One day, he had an important meeting scheduled for noon, a meeting he knew he was expected to attend. "However, as the meeting time approached, he found himself weighing the merits of attending it vs. running. When the final hour arrived, he proceeded to the dressing room, changed, departed on his run, and said, 'The hell with the stupid staff meeting.' " Morgan adds that that evening, the man was so shaken and shocked by his irrational behavior that he quit running and never resumed.

And then there is the tale of the twenty-eight-year-old school psychologist. He began by running once a day, after work, but soon he found himself running an additional seven to eight miles each morning. Then he started running in the middle of the day as well.

"I simply cannot exist any longer without a midday run," the man said. "The problem is that I am expected to counsel students throughout the day—that's my job. As I sit in my office, however, I start to become very tense and uneasy between noon and two o'clock. For the past month I have found myself going for a run in the middle of the day in addition to my morning and evening runs. I feel guilty, however, because I'm being paid to counsel students. Part of my noon run consists of my lunch period, but I always exceed that by 30 minutes or so. I know this cannot go on forever, but on the other hand I must run during midday. I know it can't go on, though—especially with the students waiting to see me—I don't know what I'm going to do."

When I ask friends and acquaintances if they've ever experienced a runner's high, I discover that some have, though usually they have kept these experiences to themselves. And I understand that—there is a limit to how crazy you want to appear.

Richard Friedman, the Cornell psychopharmacologist, tells me he had a runner's high—once. An enthusiastic athlete who swims and who used to be a runner, he says he will never forget that day.

"When I was young and foolish, I ran a marathon in the Smoky Mountains, the Nantahala Race. I have never before or since had that kind of high, and maybe it was just the result of a near-death experience."

Bill Fox said he got runner's highs "all the time." What do they feel like, I ask him.

"Did you ever do drugs?" he asked me, explaining that when he was younger he tried them all. Exercise, he said, could give him the same rush as a line of cocaine, a drug he was addicted to when he was younger. It feels exactly the same, Bill added, "except it lasts a lot longer" than the intense but momentary euphoria when cocaine affects the brain. "It's the endorphins," he explained.

I asked him to tell me when, where, and how he got those highs.

"I started to ride when I was thirty—and now I just turned fifty," Bill said in May of 2002. "But I was not riding with enough intensity, and I was still actively doing drugs." He gave up riding, gained back the weight he had lost with his exercise program, and was relatively sedentary for the next twelve years. Then he stopped using drugs, took up bicycling again, and lost weight. Two years later, he had his first exercise high. It was during a century ride—100 miles in eight hours or less. Bill's goal was to do it in under six.

"I came to a point where I had ten miles to go and less than a half-hour to do it," Bill recalled. "I had never gone ten miles in half an hour before," he said, but he began sprinting, watching his bicycle computer as it ticked off the miles and his speed, twenty miles an hour. He crossed the finish line at 5 hours, 59 minutes, and 12 seconds, completing the 100 miles with just 48 seconds to spare.

"I was high as a kite," Bill admitted. "I was totally shocked," he added, explaining that he never, ever thought that exercise could give him that feeling.

Since then, he has gotten the same high again, but it does not come easy. "You've really got to work for this high," Bill said. "To really get the effect, to really feel good, I have to ride for at least two hours at 85 percent of my maximum heart rate or for about thirty-five minutes at 90 to 95 percent of my maximum heart rate, sometimes getting up to 100 percent of my maximum." Then, he says, "I get a pretty good buzz. And it's just like with drugs. I feel on a cusp between being really high and about to throw up."

The exercise high, Bill added, "is a very similar kind of feeling to cocaine. It doesn't feel like pot, it doesn't feel like acid. It has that well-being kind of feeling, that Superman kind of feeling."

Bill noted that his exercise cravings were not cheap, explaining that he spent at least as much money on his bicycle and his gym and at least as much time and energy going after the runner's high as he spent buying and using drugs in his younger days. "It impacts my social and work life just as much as drugs did. I will turn down an invitation because that's the day I have a ride planned." He was about to start training for an annual double century—200 miles in a day—that he does with Kathryn Schwartz, the Spinning instructor at my gym, and others. It is a huge commitment, demanding training rides several evenings a week after work and long rides every weekend, alternating between New Jersey, where Kathryn and some others live, and New York, where Bill lived. The New Jersey locations are two hours by car from Bill's house. He had already told his wife that he could not accompany her on a trip to California because it would interfere with his training.

I speak to Arnold Cantor, who was fifty in 2001, when he trained for and rode the Mount Everest. He never looked like he was working too hard, cheerfully turning the pedals of his Spinning bike at a constant rate, having pushed his bike away from the fans because he does not like the chill. But it turns out that Arnold, despite appearances, is hooked by exercise-induced euphoria.

Arnold began exercising because he was concerned about his health—his father had died of a heart attack at fifty-one and Arnold wanted to avoid that fate. He joined Bally Total Fitness, a gym in East Brunswick, New Jersey, about fifteen miles from his office in Dunellen, where he is national sales manager for a company that sells lawn and garden supplies. He goes to Bally's before work to use the exercise machines.

Spinning began at Bally's at 6:00 a.m. on Tuesday, November 2, 1999, Arnold recalls. He cannot forget that moment. He had never taken a group exercise class, was not used to vigorous exercise, and, in fact, had never spent much time on a bike before, but he decided on impulse to try Spinning. That morning, he arrived twenty minutes early for the class, joining a line that would soon extend to thirty people hoping to get into a room that had bikes for only twenty. Arnold was one of the twenty and something happened to him that day that changed his life.

"I had this exhilarated feeling," he recalls. He had to experience it again, so he returned for the next class on Thursday at six a.m. The feeling came back. He was there again for a Spinning class on Saturday at nine in the morning. The next week, he was back again for the Tuesday-morning class. It became his pattern, week in and week out, three days a week, Arnold was in a Spinning class. And, invariably, he got that exercise high he craved. Soon even that was not enough. He began looking for more opportunities to spin, which is what led him to Mount Everest, and after Mount Everest, he became an instructor. Now, in addition to working full time, he teaches five classes a week—a 5:45 a.m. Spinning class on Monday mornings at Evolutions, a 6:30 a.m. Wednesday class, and one at 8:00 a.m. on Sunday in Deal, New Jersey, and the Tuesday and Thursday morning classes at Bally's. Arnold has become the instructor in the classes that got him hooked. He remains hooked. "It's just a great feeling," he said.

But Bill Fox and Arnold are extreme cases. Most people who say they exercise are more like my friend Lee Silver, a molecular geneticist at Princeton University. Lee's exercise is bike rides of about twenty miles along the packed-dirt towpath of the Delaware and Raritan Canal not far from his home. He does, however, know what it feels like to take drugs. Like Bill Fox, Lee tried a variety of drugs when he was a student in the 1970s. In his college days, Lee and a friend, an organic chemistry major, actually synthesized their own mescaline. The drug was a controlled substance but, Lee says, they traced the chemical reactions to produce it, working backward from mescaline to its roots. From that, they learned that they could buy the starting products from a chemical supply company, and that meant that they could also get absolutely pure ingredients. They bought the appropriate chemicals and took them through a precise sequence of chemical steps, ending up with their own mescaline. Lee also tried marijuana, amphetamines, and cocaine.

But the first time he experienced a runner's high it was not from exercising. "It was by doing physics," Lee tells me, and it happened in 1972, when he was a junior at the University of Pennsylvania. "I was figuring out physics for the first time, going deep into general relativity and quantum mechanics," when a feeling of ecstasy came upon him, a feeling that was just like the feeling he got when he took cocaine. "It was the same kind of high, just an incredible experience when I figured out what general relativity was for the first time," says Lee.

These days, he sometimes gets the same feeling when he exercises. "When I'm riding my bike along the canal early in the morning, and I've been riding for a few days and I'm in top shape, and nobody else is around, I get this feeling. I feel like I just want to keep going, going, going without stopping. That's what cocaine is like. It's like an extracorporeal experience. But it's not just exercise—it is exercise in a particular way when everything is working and I'm in shape and just flying down the towpath."

Lee's rides on the towpath, however, are not long nor, by my standards or by the standards of Bill Fox or my husband Bill, extraordinarily strenuous. Yet he is the sort of skeptical scientist who would never invent an experience or embellish one simply because he thought that is what someone wanted to hear. If anything, Lee would question whether there is a runner's high. So here is a new piece of information—a person who gets high without necessarily pushing his body to its limit.

Since Lee has tried other drugs, I ask him if that feeling is at all like the feeling he got with hallucinogens or marijuana. Not at all, he said. Hallucinogens altered his perceptions, making colors seem brighter, music more intense. Marijuana slowed him down, though, unlike cocaine, "it never made me feel good," Lee says. "Cocaine does not make you hallucinate. It's this very subtle feel-good kind of drug. If someone gave you cocaine and did not tell you, you might not know you were on a drug. It's not druggy—it gives you a sense that everything is perfect, like your body and mind are at their peak."

I was not much of a drug user—I never tried cocaine, although a friend in college once gave me a diet pill to try, telling me it was an amphetamine. I hated it, particularly the abhorrent compulsion I was feeling to talk and move constantly. I couldn't wait for it to wear off. Like almost everyone of my generation, I tried marijuana, smoked it at parties, but somehow it never did much for me. But I used to go along with the group, waiting for the moment when my friends announced that they had gotten the munchies, the notorious marijuana-induced food cravings. Eating was the part I liked and I enthusiastically joined in.

Yet I think I know the feeling that Bill Fox and Lee Silver were describing. I get that incredibly euphoric rush when I exercise at a very high heart rate for forty-five minutes or so, and the feeling is so wonderful that I almost can't resist going for it when I get on an elliptical trainer or when I'm in a hard, fast-paced Spinning class. It is so compelling that I often will start out telling myself I am not really in the mood for exercising and that I'll just have to force myself this time. Then the feeling clicks on and suddenly I can't stop. When I do finally get off the Spinning bike or the elliptical trainer, I still feel ecstatic for a half-hour or more, even though my heart rate plummeted down to its resting rate as soon as I stopped exercising; and not long afterward, my face is no longer flushed, I'm not sweating excessively, and there is no outward sign that I just finished a strenuous workout. Something —whether it is endorphins or some other chemicals or a combination of chemicals—seems to have changed in my brain.

Bill, however, informs me that whether I know it or not, I can seem crazy, like someone who needs a drug fix, when I get around my favorite exercise equipment. But as often as I hear about runner's highs, I hear from people who say the experience eludes them, including my husband Bill, who has exercised vigorously and regularly for more than twenty-five years.

There are others, like George Koob, a neuropharmacologist at the Salk Research Institute in La Jolla, California, who described something that sounds like the antithesis of a runner's high. Koob tells me that he used to exercise, but it usually made him feel slightly sad, rather than happy. The only part of exercise he liked was stopping. "I got to the point where I enjoyed doing it because of the relief afterwards," he says.

Steven Vogel, a sixty-two-year-old biologist at Duke University, shows up at a track three times a week, at six in the morning, and runs and walks for half an hour. "There's not a moment doing it when I wouldn't rather be somewhere else," he says. "I never get runner's highs." Yet he has faithfully kept up his program for eighteen years. Why does he do it? "It's called fear," he said. He began after he had a heart attack at age forty-three, as part of a cardiac rehabilitation program, explaining, "it seems to me that there is enough semi-objective evidence that this is a good thing to do." But Vogel is one of the very few in his program who stayed with it. Most who start, he said, stop coming after a month or two. And most who stay in, he adds, tell him that they get no pleasure from it. He thinks it is because he and the others are so slow that they never reach a physical state where euphoria can emerge. "I do ten-and-a-half-minute miles, and I'm one of the better ones," Vogel remarks.

For John Hoberman, a professor of Germanic languages at the University of Texas at Austin, the problem is not being slow. At age fifty-seven, he has been running for more than forty years, running against a stopwatch, sprinting for quarter- and half-miles, keeping it up even after an operation to replace a heart valve in 1999. Yet he, too, has never had a runner's high. He continues to run anyway, he says, for several reasons. It reminds him of his youth. He likes the spring in his legs when he takes off for a run. And, he acknowledges, "by the time I was in my forties, I definitely was out there for health reasons," worrying about his own mortality and wanting to keep his body strong.

The problem with mythologizing the elusive experience known as a runner's high, it seems, is that the feeling is unpredictable, it eludes rigorous definition, it is impossible to measure in a human being, and it is entirely unclear whether one person's high is biochemically the same event as what another person describes as a high.

Despite his own failure to feel good when exercising, Koob

tells me that he thinks there is such a thing as a runner's high and that it is different from simply feeling pleasure in one's ability to exercise. He finds it hard to dismiss all the stories from people who say they have experienced a real change in their mental state and he is swayed by the observation that some people seem to become addicted to exercise—Bill Fox said he was one of them and maybe I am, too.

The question, however, is: What is mediating this feeling? Despite the almost universal belief, outside the realm of neuropharmacology experts, that it is endorphins, Koob and others tell me they are not so sure. "It could be endorphins released in the brain, it could be dopamine, it could be serotonin. It could be almost anything," Koob confesses.

Doctors and drug users have long known about the miraculous powers of opium, including morphine, which is made from it. The great English doctor, Thomas Sydenham, wrote in 1680 that "Among the many remedies which it has pleased Almightly God to give man to relieve his sufferings, none is so universal and so efficacious as opium." But in the late twentieth century, as scientists were uncovering the biochemistry of responses to drugs and hormones (such as insulin), they began asking why people would respond to these drugs, known as opiates. It seemed too amazing to be purely coincidental that the brain just happened to undergo such a profound change, creating not just a sense of intense pleasure but also shutting off sensations of pain, just because someone smoked or injected a particular chemical from the juice of poppy seeds. The reason, many decided, must be that the opiates are mimicking a naturally occurring brain chemical. There must be some substance made by the body that mediates pleasure and pain and the opiates latch onto that system. When people take opiate drugs, they almost instantaneously flood the brain with so many of these chemicals that they overwhelm the system, inducing an opiate high.

This line of reasoning led to a search for a natural substance, the brain's own opiate.

The first clue came in 1975, when John Hughes, who was working in the laboratory of Hans Kosterlitz in Aberdeen, Scotland, found short protein fragments in the brains of pigs and showed that they could act like opiates if he injected them into the brains of animals. The next year, Roger Guillemin, a physiologist who won a Nobel Prize for his work on hormones produced by the hypothalamus, a gland at the base of the brain, reported that he had found longer opiate-like molecules in the pituitary gland. They were immensely powerful, and if they were injected into the brains of animals, the animals would feel no pain for hours. Their body temperature would drop. They would lie down, stretch out in a drug-induced stupor. To prove that the effects really were caused by a molecule that looked just like morphine, scientists showed that they could counteract them with a drug, naloxone, that completely blocks the effects of morphine.

These discoveries came at a time when scientists had learned that many hormones lock onto receptors on cell surfaces, proteins on the membrane encasing cells that serve as docking stations. Insulin, for example, attaches itself to an insulin receptor on target cells, like fat cells, muscle cells, and liver cells. Once attached, the hormone facilitates the use of glucose as an energy source, which is why people with diabetes, who either lack insulin or lack enough insulin receptors to respond to it, end up with high levels of glucose in their blood.

Scientists reasoned that just as there are receptors for glucose and other hormones, there must be a receptor for the body's own opiates. Soon, Solomon Snyder, a neurobiologist at Johns Hopkins University School of Medicine, and his colleagues found it, and an entire field of research burgeoned.

"All of a sudden, opiate receptors became a popular area," Snyder says. The chemicals were so new they had not even been named, so scientists got together to decide on one. "We had meetings to decide what to call it, and a committee decided to call it 'endorphin.' They said endorphins will include anything in the brain with opiate-like activity." (The word "endorphin" combines the first half of the word "endogenous," meaning made by the body, with the last half of the word "morphine.")

An endorphin craze began, with scientists eagerly looking for evidence that the chemicals mediated any and all sorts of pleasure. Some of the work got a little strange, Snyder says, recalling one paper in a psychiatric journal in which a scientist proposed that endorphins caused the euphoria of sexual orgasms. So he did a test on himself, to see whether naloxone would prevent the feeling.

"He sat in his room and masturbated and gave himself either naloxone or saline," Snyder says. In either case, Snyder tells me, the scientist had his orgasms. Naloxone injections "didn't make any difference," he says, and the endorphin-orgasm hypothesis went by the wayside.

At the same time, the running craze was in full swing, with enthusiasts like Kenneth Cooper, George Sheehan, and Jim Fixx singing the praises of exercise and insisting that running could change your life. "Jogging was just becoming popular in the United States and everyone was talking about the runner's high," notes Snyder. "They said, 'Well, I have a high. It must be endorphins.' "

But some scientists asked: How would you know?

The more scientists learn about endorphins, the harder that question is to answer. "In the 1970s, everyone had an idea of how simple it would be," said Roy Wise, an addiction researcher at the National Institute on Drug Abuse. Twenty-five years later, the chemicals' actions are still not well understood and researchers are still discovering new endorphins. If they fail to see an endorphin effect, Wise told me, it may be because "we have not looked at the right ones yet."

Gavril Pasternak, a neurologist who studies pain perception and opiate receptors at Memorial Sloan-Kettering Cancer Center in New York, explains one obstacle: "The problem is really a technical problem—it's very hard to define a runner's high. And then how do you quantify it? Most people describe it as not happening right away but only later on when you push yourself. And not everyone gets it every time they run," making it all the more difficult to study.

Many looked at endorphin levels in the blood and duly noted that they rise with exercise. Meaningless, scientists say. "Endorphins in the blood are irrelevant," Snyder tells me.

Huda Akil, an endorphin researcher at the University of Michigan, agrees. "What people do is they conflate the change in endorphins in the blood with what *might* be happening in the brain," she says. The problem, she explained, is no one has been able to find any evidence that endorphins in the blood do get into the brain, and yet it is endorphins in the blood that are easy to measure and the focus of most runner's-high research.

It is easy to see how the confusion arose. Scientists learned that any time a person exercises, or does anything else that stresses the body, a large precursor protein, called propiomelanocortin, is released from the pituitary gland, entering the bloodstream. It travels to the adrenal cortex, the outer layer of the adrenal gland, which cuts it into two pieces, one of which is the stress hormone ACTH (for adrenocorticotrophic hormone). Another piece is further cut up into two more fragments, one of which is known as beta endorphin.

No one knows for sure what beta endorphin does when it is released into the blood. There are hypotheses that it alters sugar metabolism or the functioning of the immune system, Akil says, but these roles are far from proven.

"This idea that when you release ACTH or when you get stressed you release beta endorphin led people to think you can do a study," Akil says. They found that beta endorphin levels in the blood do increase when people run. But, Akil stresses, "there is absolutely no evidence that it gets to the brain."

How would you know if it got into the brain, I ask her? One way would be to do a spinal tap, but that is not at all practical since spinal fluid would have to be collected while someone was running. "It is hardly the noninvasive procedure that might allow one to capture the elation of running," she says. Alternatively, researchers could do PET scans of the brain, using drugs that attach themselves to the brain's opiate receptors to determine how many of those receptors are occupied by endorphins before, during, and after a run. Once again, this is hardly practical.

A cruder method, which at least might give a hint of whether endorphins were released in the brain, would be to give runners either naloxone (the morphine-blocking drug) or injections with salt water, as a control, without telling them which substance they received. If those who got naloxone said their high was blunted, that would support the endorphin hypothesis, although, unfortunately, it would not prove it. The problem is that naloxone blocks only one group of opiate receptors, those that are used by morphine. And beta endorphin is more flexible than morphine in choosing places to bind.

There are many types of opiate receptors in the brain, Pasternak says. "The one we always think about is the mu opiate receptor—that's the one through which morphine works," he remarks. "But beta endorphin has multiple receptors through which it can act. Naloxone is very effective in blocking the mu receptors but not so effective in blocking the others."

A further complication is that beta endorphin—the one whose name is bandied about in connection with runner's high—is just one of a family of endorphins in the brain. So studying beta endorphin levels, even if it could easily be done, still would not answer the runner's high question.

"There are opiate receptors for a whole slew of these things," Akil tells me. In fact, she says, when scientists genetically engineered rodents so that they lacked the mu receptor, the animals seemed fine. It turned out that they simply switched to other receptors. "There is so much redundancy. The animals don't die—they compensate," she says.

I ask Akil and others if it is even feasible to posit that endorphins released in the brain during exercise might cause a runner's high. Akil is skeptical. The reason people get high from morphine, or other drugs, she says, is because they inject or inhale such large quantities that they flood all the brain's receptors. "An orchestrated, rapid response is required for a high." That is why children who take Ritalin, which is an amphetamine, do not get high—they take low doses, as pills, never overwhelming their brains with the drug. And, she says, "that's why it makes a difference whether you administer a drug by smoking or eating. The blood kinetics and how quickly it enters the brain are very important. We are not wired for ecstasy. We are not wired to get high. We are wired to modulate."

She is highly skeptical of the endorphin-runner's-high hypothesis. "I believe this endorphin in runners is a total fantasy in the pop culture," she says. While exercise may elicit euphoria in some people some of the time, she doubts the effect would be entirely caused by endorphins. "I think it is really simplistic to make one hormone the heart of it all. I would think it is a cocktail of goodies and that it probably is a delicate mix."

Solomon Snyder has the same reaction. "Your brain has so many neurotransmitters that influence so many different states that it could be anything."

Maybe an ability to experience an exercise high is like an ability to train to build muscle strength or endurance or to increase cardiovascular fitness—a phenomenon that can vary enormously from person to person. Maybe there are people, like my husband Bill, whose genetics prevent them from feeling this sort of euphoria when they exercise. They might be followed by people like me who can get the feeling, but only after immense effort. Then there would be people like Lee Silver who apparently can get it after what I would consider an easy workout.

This, it seems, is one of those situations where the science cannot substantiate the feeling. Yet I wonder, is it another clue to the mystery of why a few people cannot stop exercising to exhaustion while most people have absolutely no interest in such a pursuit? A few studies in rats, at least, seem to indicate that slight variations in genes can make all the difference and that addicted rats act the same way, whether their drug is morphine, cocaine, amphetamines—or running.

Lee Silver, who studied the genetic determinants of behavior in mice, likes to remind me that mice and rats have nearly all the same genes that humans do. But with rodents, there are inbred strains kept in laboratories that are exactly alike. Any two animals of one of these strains are identical twins. That makes it much easier to ask questions about genetic tendencies and genetic differences, of course, and it can point to genes that might affect human behavior.

For years, Roy Wise tells me, researchers have studied addiction in rodents, discovering that animals of one common strain, Lewis rats, are easily addicted to drugs while those of another type, Fisher rats, are more resistant. It takes Fisher rats a long time to try an addictive drug, Wise explains, probably reflecting personality differences between the strains. Once they start using the addictive drug, Fisher rats, too, become addicted. But what is truly amazing, and consistent with the notion of a runner's high, is the finding that Lewis rats are also the ones that immediately become addicted to running.

Virginia Grant, a psychologist at the Memorial University of Newfoundland, in Canada, explained how running addiction in rats works. Scientists have a set of rats that serve as controls. They are in their cages without food for twenty-three hours and then given food and allowed to eat their fill for the remaining hour of the day. The animals soon learn to eat enough in that one hour to sustain them for the rest of the day.

Another group of rats has running wheels attached to their cages for the twenty-three hours when there is no food available. Then, in the final hour, the wheels are inaccessible and the animals are offered food. Nearly all die within a week or two. They ran more each day, running twelve miles or more, running so much that it was impossible for them to eat enough during their feeding time to compensate for the calories they were expending. But instead of running less, they kept running more, and, in fact, they actually ate less than the sedentary rats. "If that is the only hour of the day when they get food, they'll starve themselves to death," Grant says.

Grant and her colleague Bow Tong Lett began investigating how similar running addictions are to drug addictions in rats. For example, psychologists have long known that rats that are addicted to drugs like morphine will learn to like the room where they had the drugs. Given a choice, they will go to the room and hang out there. So if the rats were in a room with horizontal stripes after they had morphine, they will choose a horizontally striped room over one with vertical stripes even if they had not had any drugs beforehand. But the control rats, which had never been given drugs, will show no preference for the room with the horizontal stripes.

The same thing happens with running, Grant and Lett find. And that effect, Grant adds, lets them ask how long the running high lasts. If the rats feel high when they go into the room with horizontal stripes, they will remember it and prefer it. So Grant and Lett made the rats wait for various periods of time after their run before putting the animals in the special room.

"We tried a ten-minute delay," Grant says. "We took the rats out of the wheel and put them in a home cage." Then, she and Lett put them in the special room. The rats were conditioned—they later preferred the room. But when she tried waiting half an hour before putting the rats in the special room, there was no conditioning. "The effect was gone."

Running also elicits another response that is just like one found with a drug addiction. Psychologists have discovered that rats that are addicted to morphine drink more alcohol than rats that are not addicted. Neuroscientist Stefan Brene and his colleagues at the Karolinska Institute in Stockholm find the same alcohol preference in rats addicted to running.

Addictive drugs also have a paradoxical, mysterious effect on

rats. When psychologists give rats a drink with a distinctive flavor, salty or sweet, for example, before giving them a drug like
morphine, they will subsequently spurn that flavor. Until recently,
researchers had only elicited this effect with strong drugs such as
morphine, cocaine, or amphetamine. But the same phenomenon,
Grant and Lett (as well as other researchers) find, also occurs
with running.

Rats come to like addictive drugs so much that they will repeatedly push a lever in hopes of getting them. They will do the
same thing to get access to a running wheel, Grant says.

The question is, what is going on in the brains of these rats
that makes running so irresistible? Some clues are now emerging
from Brene's lab.

The work builds on a growing understanding of the neurobi-
ology of addiction, a body of science that indicates that all addictions are, at their heart, the same. The reason is that most
addictive drugs—morphine, cocaine, alcohol, nicotine, painkillers
like Darvon, amphetamines—have a final common pathway. No
matter what else the drugs do in the brain, no matter what brain
cells they stimulate or how they affect those cells, they eventually
precipitate a chemical signal that arrives at the nucleus accumbens, a region of the brain located toward the front. And that
chemical signal often is the same—a flood of the nerve hormone
dopamine. In fact, Wise says, if you block dopamine, none of
these drugs is rewarding. Animals that used to push a lever for
cocaine, for example, to the exclusion of all else, even food, continuing until they dropped dead, will no longer do so.

"A reward is something you work for, it makes you want to go
back for more," Wise says. "It's a positive feedback in the brain
that keeps saying, 'Yes, yes, yes.' " And, he adds, while some people might crave heroin and others cocaine, others alcohol, and
others, perhaps, exercise, "the common denominator, the excite-
ment in all these behaviors is the tendency to return to them again
and again. That's what the dopamine system is for. The bottom
line is that you will like anything you can do that turns on these

dopamine neurons. And you will like anything that turns on the neurons that the dopamine neurons turn on."

The drugs that increase dopamine levels can do so in different ways. Alcohol, cannabis, and nicotine make nerve cells fire, releasing dopamine and sending it off to the reward center. Amphetamines make dopamine leak out of nerve cells, whether they are firing or not, but the end effect—a rush of dopamine into the nucleus accumbens, is the same. Cocaine has a slightly different mechanism—it stops the brain from mopping up dopamine left behind when nerve cells fire. But once again, the effect is the same, with more dopamine arriving at the nucleus accumbens.

Yes, Wise tells me, it is true that each addictive drug is said to have a different effect. Morphine makes people drowsy, it makes addicts nod off. Amphetamine users go for days without sleeping, in a state of frenetic activity. Yet those effects are, in a sense, side effects, and not the reason why people crave these drugs.

"If you talk to experienced heroin addicts, they tell you all the subjective effects of morphine. It's like a symphony," Wise says, but what makes them crave the drug is an intense, stimulating euphoria, an effect just like that of cocaine or amphetamines. "The high they are going for is all the same."

Animals, too, seem to crave a dopamine rush into the nucleus accumbens. "If you give an animal an injection of an opiate, such as heroin, it is likely to slump to the floor and not get up. But if you inject heroin directly into the part of the brain where it is rewarding, it makes the animal run around like it was given amphetamine," Wise explains. That, he says, "is the common denominator of addiction."

The dopamine that rushes to the brain's reward center is taken up by a group of cells called medium spiny neurons, and these cells, in turn, produce other nerve hormones, the small proteins, or peptides, known as enkephalin, dynorphin, and substance P.

Brene and his colleagues focused on Lewis rats, which are particularly prone to running addictions. He finds that if he gives Lewis rats free access to a running wheel, they will run about 10 kilometers (nearly 6.25 miles) a day. Fisher rats, by contrast, run only about 2 kilometers a day (about 1.25 miles). The addicted Lewis rats, Brene adds, "are more aggressive when they are denied access to the running wheels—that could resemble withdrawal from addictive drugs."

So Brene asked if running elicited the same chemical responses in the reward centers of the brains of Lewis rats as cocaine and morphine. "We know there are markers in the brain that are regulated by addictive drugs," he says. "We wanted to see if the same ones are regulated by running wheels." He looked at the production of enkephalin, dynorphin, and substance P in the reward centers of the brain. "The interpretation is that it is the same brain systems that are affected by running and by addictive drugs. It is the same brain circuitry that is activated and it is possible that you can have the same pathology in the brain, the same addictive nature of the behavior."

Brene cautions that running's biochemical effects on the brain are less than those that arise from addictive drugs. That, he says, is one reason why so few researchers have studied exercise addictions. With running, he said, "it is difficult to get clear data. It is easier to look at addictive drugs because they are so much more powerful."

The work does not reveal the initial brain signal that starts the cascade of events leading to the stimulation of the brain's reward center and the production of substances like enkephalin, dynorphin, and substance P. Perhaps, like cocaine, running prevents brain cells from reabsorbing dopamine or perhaps, like morphine, running makes brain cells fire and release dopamine. Or perhaps running has its own unique effect.

It also does not reveal the genes that make Lewis rats so addictable, ready to give up food, if necessary, to run.

But it does indicate that there may, in fact, be a runner's high, that different people might be more or less susceptible to its effects, and that the simple endorphin hypothesis does not explain the phenomenon. Bill Fox might be right that a runner's high feels exactly like cocaine—but, then, that is what one would expect of almost anything that is addictive.

Of course, euphoria is not the only effect on the brain that is touted by exercise enthusiasts. Regular exercise, many say, also combats depression, making it a natural and healthy way to deal with an extraordinarily common mental illness. I wondered what neurobiologists and psychiatric experts would say about exercise and depression.

Brene says that in his rats, running produces an increase in the same brain chemical, BDNF (for brain-derived neurotrophic factor)—as do antidepressant drugs. The chemical, which shows up in the hippocampus, a part of the brain involved in regulation of mood, is thought to be linked to relief from depression and anxiety. And, he says, when rats were prevented from running, their BDNF levels dropped.

Richard Friedman believes in exercise as part of the treatment for depression. His patients often have the worst prognoses; by the time they get to his clinic at Cornell, most have already tried the general-practitioner, take-some-Prozac route.

"I see people who are very, very severely depressed, people who are treatment resistant," Friedman says. "I make them exercise. First, I find out what they like to do—hopefully, there's something. If they don't have anything they like to do, I make them join a gym, or I tell them they have to go out walking in the morning and increase their walk each day by a couple of minutes." Patients often are taken aback, he admits. "They look at me like I'm crazy—I'm a psychopharmacologist," he explains.

Of course, he prescribes antidepressant drugs. "I've never treated anyone with exercise alone," Friedman says. But he always adds an exercise prescription to a drug prescription. "I would say that they all report that within ten minutes after stopping exercise they definitely have an improved mood and it lasts for several hours, which is much faster than antidepressants." Patients typically have to take drugs for weeks before the effects kick in.

Friedman himself is at the opposite end of the mental spectrum, one of those people who seems congenitally cheerful, always in a good mood. Yet he even notices the antidepressant effects of exercise after he works out in a swimming pool. He especially likes swimming in cold water, and speculates that it might be because the colder the water, the more it lowers your body temperature; and lowered body temperatures, for some reason, actually might improve mood. An old and venerable tradition in psychiatry was to swaddle patients in sheets dipped in ice water. "It works," Friedman says, although doctors no longer use it now that they have effective drugs. He swims in a city pool that is open for lap swimming in the morning and evening. He likes the morning, especially at the start of the season, when the water is chilly. "Not only do you work out harder, but when you're finished you have the most profound sense of relaxation," Friedman says.

But even if that is true, it sounds like an exceptional example. Most exercises raise your body temperature, yet his patients still tend to feel better after they exercise. So the temperature effect cannot be the whole story.

"Why does it work? I don't know," Friedman admits. "But people get better for hours, and those who get bitten by the bug have to keep exercising."

Despite the widespread belief in exercise's power to combat depression, it turns out that there are very few serious studies to substantiate it. One of the only ones that even attempted scientific rigor was by James Blumenthal, a psychology professor at Duke University, who compared exercise to the antidepression drug Zoloft.

Blumenthal tells me he got interested in the question after he studied the effects of exercise and yoga on mood and mental status. The subjects in that study were not depressed. Yet, he said, he noticed that there was a subgroup of people, mostly men, whose self-reported symptoms of depression lifted after they began exercising. The exercise was not vigorous—mostly easy bicycling and walking.

"We thought that if it helps nondepressed people feel better, would it have the same effect on people with clinical depression?" Blumenthal wondered. So in the late 1990s, he began a study of 156 depressed people, aged fifty and older, whom he broke into three groups, one of which was assigned to take Zoloft, the second to exercise, and the third to take the drug *and* to exercise. Once again, the exercise was mild, consisting of brisk walking, riding a stationary bike, or jogging on a treadmill for thirty minutes three times a week.

After four months, the investigators found that all the subjects had gotten better. At this point, they stopped the assigned treatments and followed their progress for six more months. At the end of that time, Blumenthal says, he noticed that exercise seemed to have a longer-lasting effect on symptoms of depression than Zoloft. Patients who had been in the exercise group and who had improved enough so that they were no longer depressed had a significantly lower relapse rate than those who had gotten better on Zoloft—a 9 percent as compared to a 30 percent relapse rate. And those who exercised on their own during the six-month period were less likely to be depressed than those who did not exercise. "We found that fifty minutes of exercise a week was associated with a 50 percent drop in the risk of being depressed," Blumenthal explains. And, he adds, "people who exercised more had a greater reduction in symptoms." But, he cautions, "we don't know if they were feeling better and therefore they did more, or if they did more and therefore felt better."

As Blumenthal readily concedes, his study does not quite prove that exercise alleviates symptoms of depression. His study had no control group that, for purposes of comparison, received no treatment. It remains possible that the test subjects might have gotten better on their own; depression is known to wax and wane, and people tend naturally to seek help when their symptoms are worse. If you simply wait four or ten months, without taking anything, might you not be as likely to get better as if you exercised?

Another problem was distinguishing the effects of exercise from the effects of social support and encouragement. The subjects who exercised did so in a group, and that itself may have helped them feel better, Blumenthal points out.

"What people really want to know is, can you simply write a prescription for them to exercise rather than take Zoloft?" Blumenthal says. The answer is, he still does not know.

And if exercise affects brain centers involved in depression, that would certainly be independent of the endorphin-runner's-high hypothesis. Depression involves a different brain chemical, serotonin, and drugs like Zoloft act by increasing brain serotonin levels.

Even those who prescribe exercise (along with medications) do not claim it is a panacea. Not everyone is helped, and some who say they feel better are still depressed.

"I did see patients who said, 'I didn't feel any better,' or, 'I felt better but it was transient,' " Friedman admits.

Friedman thinks patients have little to lose and, potentially, a lot to gain from exercise. "It's never made anyone worse," Friedman says. "Most interventions, most medicines, have lots of side effects, but I've never seen a case—ever—where a patient complains that they are more anxious or more dysphoric after they exercised. Nearly everyone who does it feels better, and no one says anything bad about it."

He also give them another piece of advice: lift weights. It will not give them a runner's high, it will not stave off depression, but, Friedman is convinced, it can give another sort of pleasure that can help anyone, his patients included, reap more joy from life. It is the pleasure of strength and power. And it is the pleasure of the actual effort of weight lifting.

Friedman is a skinny man who knows he will never build bulky muscles, no matter how hard he tries. Yet he lifts weights.

So do many women who do not want bulky muscles. How, I wonder, did this weight-lifting culture come to be? And with all the machines for working muscles and divergent advice on what works, how solid is the science behind the weight-lifting formulas? How well-founded are the beliefs that building muscle improves health, even staving off osteoporosis? How much of the weight-training advice is based on marketing and myth and how much on solid evidence?

nine

SCULPTING THE
BODY BEAUTIFUL

It was late afternoon, the end of a perfect July day in Nantucket, and the gravel parking lot at the Nantucket Health Club was starting to fill up with jeeps and SUVs. Time to work out. Eight people—five women and three men—were climbing onto bikes in the Spinning room just behind the registration desk. The small weight room downstairs was crammed with nearly a dozen men hoisting barbells and dumbbells. And next to the weight room, the wooden-floored room for exercise classes was drawing the biggest group of all, about twenty women, who had come for an hour-long class called Bodysculpting, which uses elastic bands and light weights to work the muscles.

If ever there was an illustration of the way the exercise movement has evolved, this was it—the middle-aged, affluent crowd at a Massachusetts vacation resort ending their day by lifting weights, men and women alike, trying to build, or sculpt, their bodies. When I ask why they do it, most say it is because they want to change the way they look. I understand completely, for that was what initially motivated me.

I began lifting weights in 1996, the result of a single transformative moment.

It was a chilly winter evening and my daughter Therese was in high school and passionate about lacrosse, so much that she began working with a private coach, Larry Gambrell. A few times a week, we would hear Larry's balky car with its sputtering engine pull into our driveway. Within minutes, he and Therese were in our backyard, where we had installed a lacrosse goal and set up plastic cones for running drills, or they were walking to the track of a private school nearby for more drills. Or they were on their way to the gym to lift weights. But this evening Larry was trying something different. Instead of coming to us, we were going to him, meeting him at a private high school in the Philadelphia suburbs where Larry had permission to use the gymnasium. Therese and about half a dozen other high school girls, all Larry's clients, were going to work out together. I sat in the bleachers, with the other lacrosse moms.

The girls were fast and skilled and incredibly attractive. Suddenly, I realized why they looked so good. They were not just slender and firm. They had muscles, though theirs were nothing like the image that "muscles" brings to mind. They were not bulging muscles, not even deeply defined muscles. But there was something about the muscles of their legs that gave them a shapeliness that was achingly lovely. Their calves were curved and firm and symmetrical, their thighs were slim, yet the muscles in the front and back, the quadriceps and hamstrings, were slightly rounded and subtly protruding. And their hips were slender, their abdomens flat. This is what weight lifting had done for them, I decided. It had given them strength and exquisite beauty. It's pitiful, I know, to have such thoughts—I'm the mother, for heaven's sake—but I wanted that look, too.

I wasted little time. Soon after that unforgettable night when I watched the girls practice, when Larry drove up to our house, ready to work with Therese at the gym. I asked him, would he teach me to lift? Would he design a lifting program for me? That is how I began my new life as what a fellow weight-lifting aficionado calls a gym rat. And once I learned how to lift, I came to understand the secret of the gym, that the sort of exercise that has the possibility of truly sculpting and re-forming the body is a far cry from what most women do, nor does it resemble the routines of many men who say they lift weights once in a while. It was about as far as I could get from my early days at Spa Lady, with its pink equipment and emphasis on low weights and "toning," which meant doing endless repetitions on the gym's machines, fervently hoping that we could melt away bumps and bulges and emerge firm but not obviously muscled.

When Larry and I arrived at the gym for my first session, he led me immediately into an arena that is inhabited mostly by men—the weight-lifting section, where comparatively gentle-looking machines give way to narrow benches and metal bars and racks of disk-shaped weights. In my gym, like many others, you cross into the area that is reserved for serious lifting by stepping from a carpeted area to a hard floor covered with slip-resistant rubber. There, at least back when I started with Larry, the apparatuses had yellow stickers, meant to be a joke but a bit scary, cautioning, "Warning: This Machine Builds Muscles." The walls are covered with mirrors and the mirrors have little signs on them instructing lifters not to throw their weights. It is a world with its own arcane rules of behavior and communication.

Even the way weight lifters express their agony is prescribed. I was using a leg-extension machine, in which you sit in a chair with a weighted bar across your ankles and lift the bar by pushing your legs up so they are straight out in front of you. It works the quadriceps, the muscle at the front of the thigh. And it can hurt if you pile the weight on. (Of course, no one should continue an exercise that causes sharp or sudden pain. The good pain from weight lifting is of a different sort; it builds slowly as you repeatedly lift a weight, feeling something like a burning inside your muscle.) That day, I cried out in an agony of muscle exertion, "Ooch, ooch, ooch." Larry was appalled, telling me in no uncertain terms that it was embarrassing to be with someone saying, "Ooch." The proper way to show it hurts is with a loud primordial grunt. And facial expressions must not be neglected. The appropriate one to accompany the grunting and groaning is a violent grimace.

When you load a machine with weights, Larry said, you are supposed to follow a certain protocol for putting on the plates, those disks with holes in the middle that you place on rods protruding from the machines. You're supposed to smack the plates as you add them on so that they clang with a loud ring, thus announcing that you are building a rack with some serious weights.

Then there is gym etiquette. Protocol dictates that it is selfish to hog equipment, doing endless reps (repetitions) or pyramids (sets with ever-increasing weights) while others are waiting. If you want to use a machine or weight bench and someone else is on it, you're supposed to ask, "Can I work in with you?" Then the lifter is supposed to let you do a set while he or she rests.

On the question of what to wear when lifting, it turns out that the ideal attire allows you to check your form—you want to see your entire arms and as much of your legs as possible so you can be sure that the proper muscles are contracting—although attempts to look provocative are out. Some lifters like to wear fingerless gloves, the better to grip bars of weights. Others prefer to forgo the gloves and develop calluses on their palms, a sign of serious lifting.

It was a bit like being inducted into a strange fraternity. Despite Larry's instructions, I never did break out in loud grunts, nor did I slam the weights as I loaded the machines. And I still hate it when someone wants to work in with me. But I have glimpsed another parallel world, the world of the lifters. I learned to enjoy and admire the men and the few women who lift. I learned to stride into the weight-lifting area and not be intimidated. I learned to lift weights that are heavy enough to make me strain and to love the ache in my muscles the next day and the calluses on my palms. And, of course, Larry taught me what a weight-lifting program might look like.

Over the years, I have modified Larry's program so that what I do now bears little resemblance to what I did then. I used to spend more time among the weight-lifting machines and less time in the area with the barbells and dumbbells. The machines were less threatening and seemed pretty much idiot-proof whereas the barbells and dumbbells required real attention to form. When I first tried to do a bench press, lying on my back and lowering a barbell to my chest and raising it again, I could not seem to balance the barbell—it kept tilting. When I first considered doing squats, in which you balance a barbell across your shoulders and squat down until your thighs are parallel to the floor, I decided it would be too hard. For years I used a machine instead, the Smith machine, which balances the bar for you. But there is a trade-off: squats on the Smith machine are not the same exercise. They are easier, and you do not use the subsidiary muscles that help you balance the barbell. Now I do real squats. And I do real bench presses.

Gradually, weight lifting changed the way I look. The alteration was not dramatic, but I loved it. My back became broader, which makes my hips look smaller; my arms and legs are firmer and more shapely. I never grew big muscles, but they are defined; you can see their outlines. I feel different, too, more confident of my body's strength and of my ability to do almost any movement in daily life with little effort. I know that if I stop lifting, I will lose whatever I gained, so one reason I continue with it week after week, year after year, is to keep my new appearance and my new strength. But I, like many others, continue to lift weights for another reason as well—it is a source of pleasure.

Lifting's allure can be hard to describe, as others who lift readily confess. It is nothing like the joy that comes from a hard, fast, swim, says Richard Friedman. "It leaves you with a different feeling. You have a sense of being in your body—you are aware of your body. It is like your skin has been tightened." One woman told me it is like trying to describe what it is that you like about ice cream. It tastes good, but what exactly does that mean?

John D. Fair, a competitive weight lifter who is a historian of weight lifting at Georgia College and State University in Milledgeville, says part of his enjoyment is simply that he loves being strong—he remains in awe of the way he transformed himself from a skinny, weak teenager into a powerful and muscular man. Nearly sixty years old, having lifted weights for forty years, and competed in sixty weight-lifting and bodybuilding meets, he still is drawn to gyms and keeps up a rigorous lifting program. He loves the camaraderie of lifters. "All of my good friends have been lifters. I feel a spiritual bond, a oneness with them." He also takes pride in his accomplishment. "Perhaps my greatest satisfaction comes from being able to lift as much weight as guys who weigh forty pounds more and are thirty years younger."

Exercise guru Jack LaLanne told me that, at age eighty-six, he still starts each day with an hour of weight lifting. "I do everything to muscle failure," he added, meaning that with each exercise, he lifts weights so heavy that, when he stops, he literally cannot do another repetition. "My top priority in life is my workout each day." Why does he do it? "Results," he replied. There is, as well, an aspect of personal vanity: "It's the ego in me. I want to see how long I can keep this up."

Jan Todd, the competitive weight lifter and historian of women's strength training at the University of Texas in Austin, says many women also enjoy being strong. "There is a special sense of empowerment with strength training. You don't feel as intimidated by being in a room full of men, or by many of the tasks that face us in our daily lives. Carrying groceries, carrying a child, opening heavy doors—these are things that for some women are really burdens. With strength training, a relatively small woman can see a big difference."

Then there is the pleasure of deliberately changing your body, not necessarily making it huge and bulky but making it more shapely and firm. "Strength training allows you to feel that you are in control of your body. You can make a positive change," says Todd.

That was what drew Denise Goldman, a regular at my branch of Gold's Gym, to the sport. Goldman, who was thirty-six in

2002, says she gained seventy-five pounds when she was pregnant with her daughter in 1994. She lost it by dieting and running, but after her son was born in 1999, she decided to try something different to reshape her body—lifting heavy weights. And it worked, beyond her wildest dreams. Extremely slender today, the outlines of Goldman's muscles show and give her body shape and definition. "As soon as I saw the first cuts, I was hooked," Goldman says, referring to the outlines of her muscles. "I like the look."

Even Steve Vogel, the Duke University biologist who has hated every minute of the jogging program he has followed for eighteen years out of fear for his heart's health, admits that he does not in fact dislike weight lifting. His program is not extensive—about fifteen minutes three times a week before he starts his runs. But his jacket size went from a hard-to-find size 36 to the more easily available size 38. And he discovered, to his delight, that movements that once were difficult became easy. Now he hoists his book-filled luggage onto an airplane's overhead compartment with no effort. Once, he tells me, "I just saw this dogwood tree in my front yard and I shimmied up it. Never in my life have I shimmied up a tree."

But while a program like Vogel's seems ordinary today, in fact it is very much the product of a quiet revolution in strength training. Not too long ago, weight training was seen as aberrant and extreme, even for men.

The saga of American weight lifting began in the 1930s with Bob Hoffman, a businessman in York, an industrial town in southeastern Pennsylvania, who became fascinated with strong men and big muscles. At the time, said Fair, weight lifting "had a negative image. It was practiced in sweaty gyms, dingy garages, and dirty basements by members of lower socioeconomic and immigrant groups." Fair, who published (in 1999) a scholarly study of Hoffman and his empire, *Muscletown USA*, described how Hoffman set out to convert America's men to the glories of strength training, and how he succeeded, spectacularly.

Through salesmanship and unflagging promotion of strong men and the products that, he claimed, made them that way, Hoffman dominated American weight lifting for decades. York, Pennsylvania, became known as "Muscletown, U.S.A.," and the York Barbell Company, which Hoffman founded, supplied weights to the nation's lifters. Hoffman published books, with titles such as *Broad Shoulders*, and *Big Arms*, and *Big Chest*. He also published a popular magazine, *Strength & Health*, and used it to popularize his weight lifters and another endeavor that he took up—the sale of vitamin, mineral, and protein supplements for weight lifters and bodybuilders and anyone interested in improved fitness and health. Through his unflagging enthusiasm and exuberant promotion, Hoffman ushered in the modern era, in which every gym, every health and fitness magazine, advertises and sells nutritional supplements that are supposed to improve health and enhance the effects of working out. He even had a company that sold "pure, soft water."

His story, according to Fair, is the archetypical Horatio Alger story of a self-made man of "indomitable will." Hoffman, Fair says, "was a great man, chiefly because of his capacity to promote an ideology of success."

Hoffman began by using his oil-burner factory to attract the nation's best lifters to his small industrial town. It was during the depths of the Depression and he offered champion weight lifters work in his factory, for a salary of ten dollars a week. One of Hoffman's lifters, Dick Bachtell, who had been the captain of a weight-lifting team in Hagerstown, Maryland, said he would have traveled the sixty-five miles from Hagerstown to York on his hands and knees for a job at Hoffman's factory and a chance to join his weight-lifting team.

Soon, the "York Gang," as they became known, started winning Olympic medals and bodybuilding contests. Hoffman reaped the promotional benefits. Tens of thousands of men, inspired by his ideology, "wanted to see Mecca," says Fair, and many thousands arrived over the course of four decades. His magazine, *Strength & Health*, became a bible for young men who wanted to develop and increase musculature. "It was pitched to the middle-class belief that, with sufficient willpower, anything is possible."

Fair himself practically memorized the magazines when he was first starting out. He began trying to develop muscles while a senior in high school in 1961, a lanky, gangly teenager, five feet eleven inches tall but weighing just 129 pounds. He hated his body and would wear multiple layers of shirts to make himself look bulkier. "The Charles Atlas, ninety-seven-pound-weakling thing is for real. I've been there," he said. "I wanted to be big."

Defying his parents, who were afraid he would injure himself, Fair made his own weights out of bricks and began lifting in his garage. The next year, at Juniata College in central Pennsylvania, he graduated to real weights and discovered that he could grow muscles, he could become big. "I had no natural advantages, it was just sheer determination and hard work," he explained. "The thing that fired my interest more than anything—and I have talked to countless others who had the same experience—was reading those *Strength & Health* magazines. I would read them over and over again."

Weight lifting, Hoffman stressed, was for red-blooded American men. He also promoted weight lifting for women with "Barbelles," a regular column by a woman weightlifter, but the York Gang was exclusively male. He thought of weight lifting as a way to build functional muscles, muscles that could do real work. Nevertheless, some of his lifters had extraordinary bodies, and Hoffman never tired of publishing their photographs.

One of his favorites, John Grimek, became a pin-up for men who dreamed of such a transformation. "Grimek became an inspiration to virtually all subsequent bodybuilders," Fair attests. "In his heyday, he became almost a cult figure." Vic Tanny, who went on to found one of the first chains of health clubs, was an ardent admirer who believed that "muscles will come and go but there will only be one Grimek." Steve Reeves, who won a Mr. America contest in 1947, Mr. World in 1948, and Mr. Universe in 1950 before going on to play Hercules in movies, called Grimek "the greatest bodybuilder who ever lived."

One of the most famous Grimek photographs shows him in skimpy trunks, leaning against a pedestal, his left arm flexed, right knee bent, calling to mind a statue of a Greek god. Hoffman put that photo on the cover of the September 1945 issue of *Strength & Health*. "The greatest muscle picture ever shown," he proclaimed.

Grimek and Hoffman's other poster boys also helped Hoffman hawk his nutritional supplements. At first, Hoffman had the supplement business almost to himself, and made millions of dollars in the 1950s and sixties, selling York Vitamin-Mineral Food Supplement, Hi-Proteen Fudge, Hi-Proteen Bars, and Protamin tablets, all of which, he said, facilitated the growth of muscles. His Hi-Proteen and Super Hi-Proteen supplements, in powdered and tablet forms, were his biggest moneymakers. In *Strength & Health* his champion weight-lifters were presented as evidence that his products worked. One of his weight-lifters, Jim Park, who won Mr. America, Mr. World, and Mr. Universe titles, proclaimed that he swallowed as many as two hundred Protamin tablets each day. Hoffman, who always boasted that he himself was one of the world's strongest and healthiest men, told his readers, "As for myself, I almost live on Hi-Proteen. Some days I take nothing else."

He promised that his diets and supplements would fend off aging. He published a *High Protein Recipe Book*, in which he claimed that "the shortage of protein is the greatest causative factor in aging."

By that time, in the 1960s, the Food and Drug Administration, the Federal Trade Commission, and individual scientists were questioning his products and his claims that they would build muscle and improve health, lower cholesterol, and prevent or even cure disease. Some scientists looked askance at his assertions. Philip Rasch of the California College of Medicine, for example, reported that protein supplements were no better than placebos in his studies of strength training. Hoffman struck back, criticizing the design of Rasch's study and insisting that protein supplements worked for his athletes. Rasch said he would be willing to do a larger study but that since it would require $8,000, perhaps Hoffman might underwrite it. "Unsure of the results it would produce, Bob made no such offer," notes Fair.

Despite his critics, Hoffman for the most part held his ground. One of the worst blows came in 1962, when the Food and Drug Administration made Hoffman remove his muscleman pictures from the labels of his supplements, lest customers think they might look like those weightlifters if they used the products. But he was not without his friends in Congress—for example, a sympathetic Senator Edward Long of Missouri, chairman of the Administrative Practice Subcommittee, commented: "The thought arises as to whether Quaker Oats should be required to remove the picture of the Quaker from their package, or whether the F.D.A. should mind its own business."

At nearly the same time Hoffman was building his empire in York, Pennsylvania, another movement was taking shape in southern California that celebrated athleticism and the beauty of muscular bodies for their own sake. Its home was a stretch of beach in Santa Monica dubbed "Muscle Beach," where young men and women congregated for weight training and acrobatic feats—handstands, hand-to-hand balancing, tumbling. At its peak of fame, in the 1950s, the young athletes would regularly draw thousands of admirers to the beach to watch them perform.

"The beauty of Muscle Beach was that it was so spontaneous," Fair says. "Here you had a beach with hamburger and hotdog stands. Young people put up bars and rings, they put out a platform and brought the weights out." Its proximity to Hollywood further boosted the place's glamour. When movie producers needed extras, they went to Muscle Beach to recruit young athletes. Mae West used men from Muscle Beach in her traveling troupe in the 1950s, Fair reports. "It was a strange phenomenon, even for California. It helped create the California beach culture."

It also saw the first female bodybuilders and helped launch bodybuilding as an end in itself, and gyms as a place to do it. Joe Gold, who founded Gold's Gym and then sold it and went on to found World Gym, was a regular at Muscle Beach. So was Vic Tanny, who was the first to call his gym a "health spa" and to encourage women to join. Another regular at Muscle Beach was Harold Zinkin, inventor of the Universal machine, one of the first resistance machines for gyms. Jack LaLanne came to Muscle Beach, too. Every weekend, he would drive from San Francisco to Santa Monica. A bodybuilder from his teenage years, he had even opened his own gym in 1936 in Oakland. It had separate sections for men and women and machines of his own invention. He had hired a local blacksmith to produce what he says was the first leg extension machine and the first cable pulley machine for his gym. His gym was not a success, he confesses; he told me he had to give massages to earn enough money to live on. LaLanne's national fame came from his televised exercise show that was aired from the late 1950s into the eighties.

One of Muscle Beach's most famous habitués was Pudgy Stockton, a sunny blonde who came to personify the California girl. (Her given name was Abby, which she later spelled Abbye, but she is known by the nickname she got as a chubby child.) Her boyfriend, later husband, Les Stockton, introduced her to weightlifting. At first she worried about growing too big; what she really had wanted to do was reduce. But at Les's insistence that lifting would make her more shapely, not more bulky, she developed a body that was a paragon of the Muscle Beach ideal.

"She was an absolute knockout," says Jan Todd, who has researched the history of Muscle Beach. She was also strong—she could lift Les into the air and hold him there. Yet "she was built like a showgirl. She was five feet one and 115 pounds, with a tiny waist and large breasts—very shapely." Pudgy Stockton was a poster girl, her photos as coveted and admired as those of John Grimek, the man whose body was so avidly promoted by Bob Hoffman. She was featured in photo essays in magazines, *Life*, *Pic*, and *Laff*. She was in newsreels. She was in advertisements for the Ritamine Vitamin Company and the Universal Camera Company. She was on the cover of forty-two magazines from around the world. "There were pictures of Pudgy Stockton everywhere. She was named Miss Physical Culture Venus," Todd says.

Pudgy and Les, himself a Muscle Beach star, traveled the country putting on exhibitions. She went on to open her own gym on Sunset Boulevard, for women only, and to work there as a trainer of women, Todd relates. She called it the Salon of Figure Development. To advertise it, she printed postcards with a picture of herself on the beach and stated that her gym specialized in "bust development, figure contouring, and reducing."

The phenomenon that was Muscle Beach was shut down in 1959 amidst charges that some lifters had raped young girls and that a bad element had infiltrated the area. All that is left today is a sign on the beach: "The Birthplace of the Fitness Boom of the Twentieth Century."

But in addition to giving rise to the California beach culture and the fitness boom, it also helped the marketing plans of Bob Hoffman's major rival, a Canadian entrepreneur named Joe Weider. Hoffman had largely shut Weider, and all other competitors, out of the weight-lifting business. But Weider found, and cultivated, another niche—bodybuilding, developing muscles for their beauty, not necessarily for their functionality.

Weider was a teenage wonder. Growing up in Montreal, he made his own barbells out of scrap metal and started working out. In 1939, while still a scrawny seventeen-year-old, Weider published the first issue of a magazine, *Your Physique*, which would help launch his empire. He sponsored bodybuilders, including many from Muscle Beach, and promoted bodybuilding contests for men.

"I asked myself, How many guys want to break records and how many guys want to look good?" Weider said. "For each person who wanted to compete in weight lifting, there were 100 who wanted to sculpt their body for aesthetic reasons."

He moved to Union City, New Jersey, in 1947 and began selling not just magazines but gym equipment and supplements. He boasted that he had science on his side and enlisted doctors and scientists as consultants for his magazine. One of his regular contributors was a Dr. Frederick Tilney from Hollywood, Florida, a man who had previously written for Hoffman's magazine, *Strength & Health*. Weider wrote of Tilney that he was "known far and wide as the 'miracle doctor.' " Tilney allegedly had doctoral degrees in philosophy, divinity, natural law, naturopathy, chiropractic, and food science. Weider also described Tilney as "the most forceful, dynamic, and inspiring lecturer on 'The Science of Healthful Living' in the world!"

To further promote an air of scientific credibility, Weider created a "Weider Research Clinic" at his organization's headquarters in Union City. One of Weider's own scientist-consultants, however, E. M. Orlick of McGill University, admitted that "there was no clinic as such." Fair relates that "in 1966, when Mr. America Bob Gajda visited the Weider offices, the door with the sign 'Research Clinic' led to a broom closet."

It was Orlick who conceived of a bodybuilding organization to rival the Amateur Athletic Union, the weight-lifting organization controlled by Hoffman. In 1947, Joe Weider and his brother, Ben, founded such a group, the International Federation of Body Builders.

But mostly Weider promoted muscular bodies, both male and female. He sponsored bodybuilders, he showed them off in his magazines, a publishing empire that eventually grew to include *Muscle & Fitness*, *Muscle & Fitness Hers*, *Flex*, *Men's Fitness*, *Shape*, *Fit Pregnancy*, and *Natural Health*. He created the Mr.

Olympia contest. He started a company, Weider Nutrition International, Inc., in Salt Lake City, to market products that, he claimed, would enable people to build sculpted bodies, and he sold bodybuilding books and videos.

Weider was Hoffman's nemesis. Hoffman relentlessly fought the notion that bodybuilding could be an end unto itself and mocked bodybuilders' exercises to develop a triangular-shaped upper body. The Amateur Athletic Union formulated rules for bodybuilding contests that required that the men have athletic ability in addition to muscles. "You had to have an affadavit from a high school football coach or a letter jacket. You had to demonstrate your athleticism," Todd notes.

In his magazine, Hoffman wrote witheringly about men who would simply build muscles to look good: "A *boobybuilder* is usually a young man who has nothing better to do with his time than to spend four or five hours a day in a small gym doing bench presses and curls and lat pulley exercises. He usually wears his hair long and frequently gilds the lily by having it waved. He lives for his big moment when he can strut and posture under the glare of a spotlight before an audience of several hundred followers of his peculiar cult."

Weider fought back, attacking Hoffman in his magazine, until, at one point, in 1958, their battles erupted in court. Hoffman wrote that Weider was a rat, a skunk, a jackal, a hyena. Weider sued him for libel. But Hoffman countersued Weider for malicious conspiracy and character defamation. Finally, in 1965, the lawsuits were settled—Hoffman won, and the court awarded him the sum of one dollar.

In the end, however, after years of battling Hoffman, Weider prevailed. Bodybuilding became more popular and the sport of weight lifting declined. The reasons, sport historians say, had to do with changing fashions and with American weight lifters' fall from grace.

In the 1960s, Americans, including Hoffman's lifters, began losing in Olympic events. Soon the specialized sport of Olympic lifting, which America, and the York gang, had dominated for decades, and which had drawn thousands of men like Fair to weight lifting, began losing its allure. Even the classic Olympic lifting movements fell out of favor.

Three precisely defined movements had been part of the Olympics since the 1928 games in Amsterdam. They are three difficult maneuvers known as the press, the snatch, and the clean and jerk, always done in that order.

To do the first competitive lift—the press—the athlete begins by "cleaning" the barbell—leaning over, squatting down, and pulling the bar upward so rapidly that it does not stop until it is resting on the lifter's shoulders. Once the bar is on the shoulders and the lifter has regained his balance, the referee gives a signal for the lifter to begin the official "press" overhead during which the lifter is not supposed to bend his legs or lean over backward in any way.

With the snatch, the weight lifter, using a wide-spaced grip, pulls the bar up from the floor. As it nears its peak, he ducks under it and catches it with his body in a squatting position under the weight, arms outstretched. When the lifter with the weight is stabilized in the low position, he stands up with the weight and holds it over his head. In the clean and jerk, the lifter again begins by cleaning the weight. However, because the weights in this lift are so much heavier than those used in the press, elite lifters learned to drop rapidly into a deep squat or a front-to-back split so that the barbell does not have to be pulled so high. Once the barbell is on the shoulders, the lifter comes out of the squat or split until he or she is standing upright. Then, with a vigorous half-squat and thrust, the barbell is thrown overhead to arms' length. As the weight nears its peak, the lifter ducks under it and catches it while he is in a low position with his elbows locked. In a final movement, he raises himself and the weight so that he is standing erect with the weight overhead. Any pressing of the weight is cause for disqualification.

In competition, a lifter does each lift three times and his score is the sum of the highest weight he can lift in each movement. The winner is the man with the highest total score.

In 1972, the press was eliminated from the Olympics because, Fair explains, lifters were cheating so rampantly, flouting the rules by using their hips and back to lift the weight, and getting away with it, that it seemed best to get rid of the move altogether. "That took the heart out of the sport," says Fair. "In the 1950s, the standard question was, 'How much can you press?' Now, no one does overhead lifts anymore. I do them sometimes in the gym, and people look at me like I'm a dinosaur."

"What had enabled Hoffman to remain paramount in body-building and powerlifting was the loyalty of the weight-lifting clique that controlled the AAU power structure," said Fair, referring to the Amateur Athletic Union, which sponsored weight-lifting competitions. "With the decline of Olympic lifting, however, the ground started to shift."

Yet Weider's victory and the triumph of bodybuilding came at a cost, Jan Todd asserts. Hoffman's battles with Weider had in-cluded a smear campaign that succeeded in tainting the sport. It became known, she said, as something for "the funny guys who just care about their biceps." Fair knows that era well. While he was proud of his newly muscular body in the 1960s, he also was a bit ashamed of lifting. In those days, it was associated with gay men and men who were, he said, weird. "The people who did it wore tight shirts. They liked to show off their muscles. I was al-most embarrassed to be lifting weights."

Hoffman successfully advanced the notion that bodybuilding was connected to the world of homosexuals, Todd notes. "That stuck and has continued to this day. In the 1960's, you had to be a very brave man to be involved in a sport like men's bodybuild-ing. There were issues that could be raised."

At the same time, there was, as William Kraemer, an exercise physiologist at the University of Connecticut who studies weight training, puts it, "the dark side of the sport"—steroid use. "Obviously, drug use was against the cultural norm," Kraemer says. It gave weight lifting and bodybuilding an unsavory air.

Steroids were developed in the 1930s and were originally used to help build bodies of the weak and elderly, among other things. They were rediscovered by Russian weight lifters in the late 1950s. At first, Hoffman's lifters were leery of trying them. A doctor, John Ziegler, tried to get Grimek to take them in 1959. "He gave me one of those half-bushel baskets with the pills to try and get some of the lifters to try them," he told Fair. "No one would."

Their reluctance gave way to acceptance when they began losing to the Russians and decided that the steroids would increase their strength. In 1971, one of Hoffman's lifters, Ken Patera, crowed to reporters about how he could not wait for the 1972 Olympic Games so that he could compete against Vasily Alexeev, the Russian who had beaten him in the World Championships. "Last year, the only difference between me and him was that I couldn't afford his pharmacy bill. Now I can." Come Munich, he added, "we'll see whose steroids are better, his or mine." (Alexeev won again in '72, however, and Patera, defeated, turned to professional wrestling.)

That same year, Hoffman's *Strength & Health* published an editorial by Bill Starr, a weight lifter who was the magazine's associate editor, in praise of the drugs: "Some go so far as to say that it is immoral to use anabolics [i.e., anabolic steroids]. It should be considered cheating and any drug use should be banned. Yet, anabolics are being used by just about everyone in this sport." Starr added that "the only immorality in my mind on the entire subject of anabolics is keeping it secret."

Many readers were furious, writing letters decrying the corruption of the sport. Hoffman fired Starr but replaced him with another lifter, George Lugrin, who continued to encourage an openness about the drugs, writing in an editorial that while the outrage over Starr's editorial was "predictable," it really should be no surprise that the drugs were in use. "Those on the 'inside' knew. And those on the 'outside' didn't want to know. Nonetheless, it shouldn't have been shocking to discover that science and technology had scaled the victor's stand."

Steroid use continued, and flourished. Terry Todd, a historian of weight lifting at the University of Texas at Austin—and Jan Todd's husband—was a weight lifter with Hoffman's York Gang in the 1960s. Now he crusades against them. In the 1980s, he reports, one California doctor, Walter F. Jekot, was flagrant enough to pass out fliers that made the following offer: "Bodybuilders— For each new patient you refer to our office you will receive one of the following: 1. Either six free Deca 50 mg. Injections or three free Deca 100 mg. Injections." The drug, decadurabolin, is a derivative of testosterone. (In 1993, Jekot was sentenced to five years in prison for dispensing steroids and human growth hormone to athletes.)

Since it is illegal to use massive doses of steroids in an attempt to increase muscle size and strength, there are no scientific studies in humans of what happens when healthy people take huge doses. But it is clear that with steroids weight lifters became noticeably bigger and stronger.

As for women, they never really took to bodybuilding or weight lifting. While magazines like *Strength & Health* and *Ironman* were full of stories about women lifters, "for the most part they were working in isolation," according to Jan Todd.

Todd broke into the sport in the seventies, largely as a result of her marriage to Terry Todd, who became her coach.

Born in 1952, her only previous foray into athletics was as a member of her high school swim team in Plant City, Florida, in her freshman and sophomore years. Then, she says, "I gave it up because it wasn't cool." But shortly after college, when she married Terry and found herself tagging along when he went to gyms, she decided to try lifting for herself. At first she did what many women do today—lots of reps at low weights. But, she says, "I found it really tedious and boring." She decided she could do much more.

"I got caught up in this quest for strength. I was just drawn to this notion of seeing how much I could lift." She did a little research and found that the women's record for deadlifting—bending over and hoisting a weight-laden barbell to mid-thigh with the body fully erect—was set in 1926 by a professional strongwoman, Jane DeVesley, who lifted 392 pounds. "I started out with this harebrained idea that it would be cool to get into the *Guinness Book of World Records*. It was fun and it was something to do while I tagged along with Terry." She was certainly an oddity in gyms, where few women ventured, but she discovered that she had an unrealized genetic gift: she could get very strong.

In 1975, Todd attempted to enter her first meet, a powerlifting competition. "I was told that I could not compete because I was not a man. So I had to give an exhibition." All the men finished competing, and then she did her lifts, breaking the previous world's record for women by deadlifting 394.5 pounds. A year later, she deadlifted 412 pounds.

In November of 1977, *Sports Illustrated* wrote about her in an article, "The Pleasure of Being the World's Strongest Woman," and for years afterward, the moniker stuck.

It was not until the next year, in Nashua, New Hampshire, when a women's powerlifting meet was held for the first time, that Todd finally was an official competitor. She broke the women's record again, deadlifting 453 pounds.

She became a celebrity, appearing on national TV programs, such as Johnny Carson's *Tonight Show*, where she deadlifted 415 pounds five times in a row. Johnny tried but failed to pick up the weight, and only when he was assisted by the actor Carl Reiner and Jack Klugman, star of the television show *Quincy*, could he manage to lift it.

Despite Todd's fame, women were still unwelcome in the weight-lifting world. Meet organizers sometimes said it was fine for a woman to enter, but she had to abide by the same rules as men. Todd tells of humiliations: "The rules stipulated that you had to wear a jockstrap and you had to weigh in in the nude. Some recalcitrant judges would say, 'You can't lift in my meet unless you wear a jock, and you can't wear a bra, and you have to weigh in in the nude in front of men.' "

Women came to steroids later than men, but by the end of the eighties, female bodybuilders and weight lifters also were pumped up with the drugs. Most kept mum about their drug use, but observers were certain that the women could never have gotten so muscular without steroids. One woman, however, Tammy Thompson, spoke to Terry Todd in a recorded interview on April 15, 1986.

"I remember after my first powerlifting meet thinking, 'I can't believe I finished sixth out of the nine women in my weight class. I know I'm stronger than they are.' " She was certain the other women were taking drugs, and so she would, too. Soon, she said, she was taking a full course of steroids, increasing her doses as her meet dates approached.

"How did I feel? Like I was on the top of the world. Not high, just a very super feeling. I thought I could do anything." Eventually, her voice deepened, "and I noticed these strange hairs showing up. I thought, 'Well, that's no big deal. A hair here, a hair there. Big deal. I can live with it.' Some of it was on my face, some on my chest. And the next cycle it got worse. But by then, I figured the damage had already been done, and I went ahead with the full cycle of steroids because I had a meet coming up. It's hard to explain to people that once you're on the drugs you lose sight of everything but winning . . . I could sort of see what was happening and I didn't care." At the time of the interview, she said, she had not taken steroids for two years, "but I still have to shave every day."

Women who lifted weights and competed in bodybuilding contests began to appear more and more extreme, achieving bodies that few other women aspired to. In 1981, NBC sports announcer Mike Adamle told Jan Todd that although the public might want to see female weight lifters *once*, as they might want to see sideshow freaks, there would never be a continuing audience for their sport.

"Women's bodybuilding is in decline," Todd now says. "We were painted into a corner by not getting in control of the drug issue. Women bodybuilders are so large and so muscular and so unusual looking that it's just too fringe."

Outside the small world of weight lifting, strength training used to be frowned upon, for women *and* men. When Ken Cooper and the aerobics movement emerged in the late 1960s, exercisers were specifically advised not to lift weights. They were told there was no reason to add bulk when what they wanted was speed. "Muscular fitness is of some value, but it is too limited," says Cooper in his book *Aerobics*. "It concentrates on only one system of the body, one of the least important ones, and has limited beneficial effect on the essential organs or overall health. It's like putting a lovely new coat of paint on an automobile that really needs an engine overhaul. Endurance fitness should be your goal."

Likewise, lifting had no place in the jogging movement spearheaded by Jim Fixx and George Sheehan.

In fact, says Jan Todd, weight lifting was even discouraged by many of the entrepreneurs who advertised in muscle-building magazines. Starting with Charles Atlas in the 1920s, the strength trainers whose businesses were based on mail order needed to focus on exercises that did not require large and heavy apparatus. "In the 1960s, there was a big boom in expander exercises, springs and cables, something cheap and inexpensive." Charles Atlas had started that trend. He had been an artist's model—his given name was Angelo Siciliano—who came to fame after winning a contest, held by Bernarr Macfadden in 1921, "America's Most Perfectly Developed Man Contest."

In promoting his mail-order training business, Atlas claimed that he developed his body without lifting heavy weights. Others disputed him and Hoffman took Atlas on publicly, stating, "I can prove through a hundred sources that he trained with weights." Fair says he knows people who personally observed Charles Atlas training with weights. Still, the belief persisted that weight training was unnecessary.

Yet the Muscle Beach crowd and the gyms they started, the York Barbell Company and the equipment it sold, Weider and his magazines and bodybuilding contests—these had laid the groundwork for today's strength-training movement. What was needed was an impetus for ordinary people to decide to lift weights.

The impetus came from several directions and it led to a profound change in the interest of scientists in this pursuit, which had long been almost exclusively the domain of marketers.

For men, says Fair, the negative image of bodybuilding started to dissipate with the advancement of Arnold Schwarzenegger in the 1970s. Joe Weider sponsored him, bringing him to America from Europe, posing him in Gold's Gym in Santa Monica and putting him on the cover of *Muscle Builder/Power* in July of 1968 (in 1980, the magazine was renamed *Muscle & Fitness*). Schwarzenegger won bodybuilding contest after contest—Mr. Olympia, Mr. Universe. He became a movie star. He married into the Kennedy family.

"Arnold was big and strong and he was terribly engaging," Fair says. He had a modest demeanor, he seemed almost amused by himself. He was charming, he was likable. With him as a model, weight lifting became acceptable. But, I comment, Arnold was so big. "That's what guys want," Fair replies.

Another change came when exercise physiologists discovered that, contrary to what coaches had believed, weight training could improve athletic performance. The thought used to be that athletes would become "muscle-bound," strong but slow. Jan Todd said that idea emerged in the nineteenth century, by analogy with horses. Draft horses were muscular and slow, but athletes wanted to be more like sleek racehorses, it was said. "A man who would build larger muscles would make himself into a human draft horse," Todd explained.

Jack LaLanne said that when he opened his gym in Oakland in 1936, athletes had to sneak in. "Their coaches said they would get muscle-bound. I gave them keys to go in at night."

It was not until the seventies that athletes, discovering they could gain a competitive advantage, began regularly, and openly, lifting weights. Soon even high school athletes were venturing into weight rooms.

Almost simultaneously, in the late seventies, the health-club movement, which grew out of the aerobics movement, saw a marketing opportunity. Clubs began advertising classes that promised to sculpt women's bodies, along with personal trainers to help clients, men and women, learn to lift weights. Gyms attracted clients with a promise of the newly fashionable lithe and strong bodies, the sort that were starting to show up in Hollywood.

The allures of strength training were on display when, in 1982, John Travolta reshaped his body for the movie *Stayin' Alive*. Other stars soon approached his trainer, Dan Isaacson, among them Linda Evans, Burt Reynolds, and Jack Nicholson. Another trainer, Jake Steinfeld, worked with Harrison Ford to shape his body for the role of Indiana Jones. Linda Hamilton, in the 1992 movie *Terminator 2*, displayed a muscular body with a wide back that could only have come from lifting weights.

For women, an impetus was the passage of Title IX, the 1973 law that required that universities receiving federal funds provide women with equal access to athletic facilities. Todd was an undergraduate at Mercer University in Macon, Georgia, that year. "Women were not allowed in the weight room," she recalled. "After Title IX passed, we could get in the door. Women began to see weights used to help athleticism."

Health clubs emerged in nearly every town: Gold's Gym,

World Gym, Vic Tanny, 24 Hour Fitness, New York Sports Club, Bally Total Fitness, Reebok Fitness. Their appeal was boosted, Kraemer says, by the introduction of equipment other than barbells and dumbbells, which can seem rather intimidating. A host of inviting weight-training machines—including the pink ones at my original gym, Spa Lady—were designed with the specific object of drawing clients in.

Along with the new interest in weight training came a new interest in the science of building muscles. Some weight lifters, like Richard Berger, an emeritus professor at Temple University, and Patrick O'Shea, an emeritus professor at Oregon State University, were originally drawn to lifting by the likes of Weider and Hoffman, and only later became scientists to study the foundations of their sport. Other academic researchers were simply intrigued and began questioning old assumptions about building muscles, seeking to distinguish what was myth and what was reality.

One of the old beliefs of weight trainers and exercise physiologists was that you got stronger when your muscles grew larger. It made sense—the men who had lifted weights developed large muscles and, as anyone who has had a leg in a cast can attest, a muscle that is not used shrinks and weakens. But as women started entering weight rooms, the exercise physiologists who studied them were struck by the way they could grow strong but not big. Women, Costill and Wilmore report, can have the same percentage strength gains as men—getting 25 to 100 percent stronger within three to six months—yet their muscles often grow no larger. But how could that be? And what determines whether muscles grow big, strong, or both?

Cardiologist and marathon runner Paul Thompson, of Hartford Hospital, decided to investigate. He had spent most of his adulthood asking questions about exercise. He was one of the first athletes ever to travel to Ball State University to have Dave

Costill biopsy his muscle as part of a research project. And he was intensely curious about his own inability to develop large muscles. A skinny man, with a typical distance runner's body, Thompson lifted weights, yet his muscles never grew much bigger. He suspected there was a strong inherited tendency for muscles to respond, or not respond, to weight training.

"Some people get big just by walking by the barbells," Thompson says. "Others can lift weights a lot and their muscles don't grow much."

Thompson, along with Eric Hoffman, a geneticist at the Children's Hospital Medical Research Center in Washington, D.C., and others around the country recruited 700 men and 700 women who had not previously lifted weights. These volunteers agreed to train the biceps and triceps muscle of their nondominant arm in a laboratory, leaving their dominant arm untrained for comparison. Their muscle size before starting to train was measured with an MRI scan, and their muscle strength was ascertained by a device that measures how much weight they can push in one attempt with their triceps, at the back of the arm, or pull with their biceps muscle, at the front of their arm.

It immediately became clear that although muscle size and strength appear to go together, they are, in fact, independent. Some people can gain size but not strength and others can gain strength but not size. Some gain both; a few gain neither. It is much like aerobic training, where there seems to be a sort of bell curve of responsiveness; some quickly gain muscle strength or size, and others are fated never to progress, no matter how hard they try.

If muscle genes are the key to individual variations in the ability to build muscle size or strength, there should be differences in these genes that might determine who gets big, who gets strong, who gets both, and who gets neither.

But at the same time, Hoffman believes, the work raises ethical questions. Should people be told if they have genes that will prevent them from getting stronger or from growing larger muscles? Should coaches do genetic testing of athletes to decide who are the best candidates for a team? Should teenagers interested in such sports as football and wrestling be able to learn their genetic potential?

It is a gray area, barely studied because until now almost all the research on genetic testing and its psychological effects has focused on more profound questions, like—Who should be tested for genes that predispose to breast cancer? Should people be offered tests for genes that increase the likelihood that they will develop Alzheimer's disease? Should children be tested to see if they inherited genes for diseases such as Huntington's, which usually occurs in middle age?

Erynn Gordon, a genetic counselor in Hoffman's group, says the muscle study will specifically address the testing issue. Each subject took a psychological test, a self-concept assessment, before the research began, she explains. When the study is completed, they will be informed of their genetic profiles and will take the self-assessment test again, allowing investigators to compare their self-images before and after getting the news.

While some researchers, like Paul Thompson, always suspected that muscle size and muscle strength need not go together, some of the other assumptions about weight training are so deeply held that to question them is to risk disbelief.

Does weight training stave off osteoporosis? No one really knows, says J. Christopher Gallagher, an osteoporosis researcher at Creighton University, in Omaha, Nebraska. It is true that weight lifters, in general, tend to have denser bones, but is that because they lift weights or is there some other genetic factor that leads to both an ability to gain muscle and bone density when you lift weights? Osteoporosis, after all, is a disease, not simply a matter of less dense bones. It is characterized by bone fractures. What is needed is a study showing that people who were randomly assigned to lift weights had fewer fractures than another group who, for comparison, were not assigned to lift weights. No study has ever shown that.

Still, Gallagher asserts that weight training is beneficial for people with osteoporosis because it strengthens muscles, improving stability and making bone-breaking falls less likely.

A group of medical experts convened by the National Institutes of Health to examine evidence on the prevention, diagnosis, and treatment of osteoporosis came to that conclusion. In a paper published in 2001 in the *Journal of the American Medical Association*, the group, chaired by Anne Klibanski, a professor of medicine at Harvard, wrote: "Randomized clinical trials of exercise have been shown to reduce the risk of falls by 25 percent, but there is no experimental evidence that exercise reduces fracture rates."

I ask a simple question, about an article of faith among exercisers. Muscle burns more calories than fat, we're always told. So, I want to know, if you do resistance training the way most of us—not the professional weight lifters—do it, will you noticeably increase your body's metabolism?

Sorry, says Claude Bouchard, the researcher studying the genetic inheritance of the ability to train. Weight lifting has virtually no effect on resting metabolism. The reason is that any added muscle is minuscule compared with the total amount of skeletal muscle in the body. And muscle actually has a very low metabolic rate when it is at rest, which is most of the time. Skeletal muscle burns about 13 calories per kilogram of body weight over twenty-four hours when a person is at rest. A typical man who weighs 70 kilograms (or 154 pounds) has about 28 kilograms of skeletal muscle, Bouchard says. His muscles, when he is at rest, burn about 22 percent of the calories his body uses. The brain would use about the same number of calories, as would the liver. If the man lifts weights and gains 2 kilograms (4.4 pounds) of muscle, his metabolic rate would increase by 24 calories a day. According to Jack Wilmore, the exercise physiologist at Texas A&M, the average amount of muscle that men gained after a serious weight-lifting program that lasted twelve weeks was 2 kilograms. Women, of course, will gain much less.

I saw the problem when I looked at a chart in Vogel's book on muscle showing how much blood is delivered to various parts of the body at rest and during exercise. The more blood delivered, the more metabolically active the cells are and the more calories they are burning. At rest, skeletal muscle gets 1.04 liters of blood each minute, about a fifth of the blood being pumped through the body. The rest goes to places like the digestive system (1.20 liters per minute), the kidneys (0.95 liters), and the brain (0.64 liters).

During intense exercise, the skeletal muscles get a huge increase in their blood supply, with 17.6 liters each minute arriving to fuel them and give them oxygen. Then, 88 percent of the body's blood is going to the muscles, taken mostly from the digestive system and the kidneys. So it looks as if skeletal muscles are not really doing much except during those brief periods of exercise, and it would take a lot of muscle to substantially increase the body's metabolic rate—much more than most of us will ever build in our workouts at the gym. To burn more calories, it seems, requires more intense exercise, like running, and not just putting on some muscle and hoping it will burn calories and make you thinner as you rest.

A corollary to the hypothesis that you will burn more calories simply by adding some muscle is the fervent belief that your body weight is not so important when you are lifting weights. The idea is that when you do resistance training, you may lose some fat, but you won't necessarily weigh less—you may weigh the same or a little more—because you're building muscle at the same time. There is a grain of truth there, since muscle weighs more than fat. But, Bouchard cautions, the problem is that almost no one puts on enough muscle as a proportion of their total body mass to make a noticeable difference in their weight. The idea that you will weigh the same or more but you really are thinner is just another exercise myth.

Bouchard doesn't want to discourage people from building

muscle. The muscle you develop, he emphasizes, is more efficient, with more mitochondria and it is better at using fat for fuel. The cells also are more permeable to glucose, which, in turn, reduces the need for excess insulin in the blood. The result is a reduced susceptibility to diabetes. But it would be unreasonable to expect that you can eat more because, after all, your metabolism has gone up with more muscle mass and that even if your weight goes up, that's okay because you really are thinner.

I try another question: Why do muscles get sore? You will feel fine when you are lifting or when you are doing something like hiking down a mountain. But a day or two later, your muscles start to ache.

Larry Rome thinks he knows the answer. It is generally accepted that when muscles do eccentric contractions—lengthening as they generate force, like quadriceps muscles when you walk downhill—they are put under unusual stress. The chains of molecules that make up muscle fibers may snap. "It's this business about the weakest link. The weakest can sometimes pop." It is probably either these submicroscopic tears or the subsequent muscle inflammation that causes delayed pain.

Others, like Stanley Salmons, remain skeptical. He agrees that eccentric muscle contractions are more likely to cause muscle damage, but that isn't necessarily the source of delayed soreness. "Damage and pain have different time courses, and they respond differently to repeated bouts of exercise. At this moment I do not know why muscles get sore and no one else does either."

Does stretching before or after exercise help prevent soreness? "You hear trainers say it's very important to stretch before exercise," Salmons says. "But there were experiments in which people did exercise with or without stretching and it didn't seem to make much difference." But, he says, it does seem to help if you start your exercise gradually, warming up by jogging before starting to sprint, for example. "Warming up the muscles before exercise definitely does seem to have a beneficial effect," he asserts.

What about taking an anti-inflammatory drug that also relieves pain, like ibuprofen? A pain reliever, like ibuprofen, can make people feel better, but whether it speeds healing is an open question.

In the meantime, most of us simply assume that if we start to work our muscles, something will happen—our bodies will change in shape and maybe in size. The problem, some weight-lifting experts say, is that many people follow lifting programs that are destined to fail, and that is a particular problem with many of the programs that are promoted for women.

"From the time of Vic Tanny on, women who went to gyms wanted to work on their appearance," Todd says. "What we now perceive of as toning is in large part an offshoot of the aerobics boom. It was about creating bodies that were lean, slender, and not really very muscular. That carried over into lots of repetitions with low weights."

Jane Fonda, for example, told women to do sixteen repetitions of exercises, like circling their arms, with no weights. In her "advanced exercises" she suggested strapping half-pound or one-pound weights to the wrists and repeating exercises like arm circles thirty-two times. Such a program, alas, does little, though the selling point for gym owners is that it is safe. "To teach someone how to lift properly takes time," Todd says. It is so much easier to give clients a routine that will not hurt them and that can make them believe they are toning their bodies. But the results are predictable. "The sad thing is that they don't see many results, so they quit."

Kraemer, who is the editor of one of the leading strength-training publications, the *Journal of Strength and Conditioning Research,* says one reason women start such programs is that they are afraid to lift weights that seem heavy, worrying that weight lifting will give them the muscles of men.

"Women have been sold a myth of becoming big. They don't have the genetics." Even women who are genetically capable of growing big muscles can never grow muscles as large as those of a man. Kraemer biopsied the muscles of women bodybuilders who spent hours each day lifting weights. "They had smaller muscle fibers than the average male," he says. "And these were women who were taking drugs" to increase their muscle mass.

"A lot of women say, 'I won't lift a heavy weight,'" Kraemer tells me. "They're just sitting there with ten-pound weights. "It's better than zero, but they're taking a second-class program. If we told you that in business you would have to take a second-class program, that would be considered prejudicial." The result, Kraemer insists, is that most women "dramatically undercut themselves."

He also says that it is futile to try to spot reduce—working your inner thighs, for example, in hopes of slimming them. "Spot reducing is not a real thing," Kraemer says. Nevertheless, he says, "bodysculpting relates back to the fact that while you cannot spot reduce fat you can spot increase the size of a muscle with specific strength training. The term has come out of the fitness-marketing people and bodybuilding community." As for toning, "It is a highly ambiguous term in the fitness world," something that cannot be physically measured." It is "a gestalt of many factors that can be defined and viewed differently by different people, but it is more a visual perception of muscle fitness and firmness."

With so many people trying to lift weights, is it reasonable to expect that they will look better? It is possible, Kraemer says, but, "to reshape yourself, you have to hypertrophy muscles," meaning you have to build them. That can take time—three to six months of concerted effort or even longer, Kraemer asserts. And not everyone can get a body that would qualify as "toned." That depends on whether one is genetically capable of building muscle and whether one is thin enough for the muscle to show.

As anyone who has ever started a lifting program soon realizes, it can be hard to sort through weight lifting's long and contradictory list of rules and prescriptions. You can't work the same body part two days in a row. You have to do three sets of about ten reps, meaning you should repeat an exercise ten times, take a break, repeat that set again, take another break, and repeat the set again. No, some say, you do better with four sets. Some advise twelve reps. Others insist that the way to lift is to do one set to failure, meaning you should make the weights so heavy that after about six or eight repetitions you literally cannot do another one. Then you move on to another muscle group. What is the evidence for the different protocols? And how should people plan a lifting program?

Scientists, through repeated studies, have discovered some general principles. "We know a lot," Kraemer said. Investigators learned that people must stress muscles with weights that are challenging in order to elicit increases in strength or size. The order of the exercises is important: they should work large muscles, like those of the quadriceps, before small muscles, like those of the inner thigh. That is because working a small muscle first fatigues the adjacent larger one. The main variables in a weight-lifting program, he said, are intensity, resistance, order, and choice of the number of sets. The lifting exercises also should vary, so a person does not do exactly the same thing week after week, month after month. By manipulating those variables, people can achieve their goals.

The accumulated knowledge to date is published in a position statement that Kraemer and a committee he headed wrote for the American College of Sports Medicine. The paper, which appeared in 2002, is impressive. If it has one theme it is that a variety of programs are effective but you have to keep stressing your muscles if you want to see any change. On specific questions, though, it often equivocates, noting that the details of a program depend on one's goals and that some questions still cannot be answered.

Should you do one set or several? Studies have not answered that question, it says. Should you use free weights, like dumbbells and barbells, or machines? Beginners and intermediates should use both, and advanced athletes should spend most of their time with free weights but also should use some machines. What about the speed with which you perform your weight-lifting exercises? It is important to train at fast, moderate, and slow speeds, the paper says. But the most effective speed seems to be about one second to one to two seconds for a contraction and about the same for a muscle lengthening.

The paper says you should train every major muscle group of your body two to three days a week but that if you are at a stage where you work on one body area (say, the upper body) in each session, you should work that body area just one to two days a week.

Kraemer tells me that if there is one overarching message for weight lifters it is that they must vary their training, changing their routine to do different exercises, with fewer or more repetitions, lighter and heavier weights, to see results and also to stay motivated. "A beginner may do one set of eight to twelve repetitions, but you can't do this the rest of your life. You'd be bored out of your mind."

Yet many who lift weights actually resist learning what science has to say, Kraemer observes.

"Weight training is mythology for some people. They don't like science and they deal with beliefs that have nothing to do with facts." In addition to studying weight training, Kraemer also does peptide research, studying small fragments of proteins. Needless to say, people respond very differently to that aspect of his work. "When I do peptide research, no one is going to tell me, 'I don't believe that happened,' whereas with weight training, people will tell me that. It's got its own culture. And people are very visceral about what they believe. That ties into the marketing."

If you want to market a program, why bother to do a scientific study? It turns out to be easy to devise new exercise programs and promote them, regardless of objective evidence. Kraemer and a colleague once calculated how many possible ways there were to do a weight-lifting program, varying the order the muscles are worked, and the particular exercises for each muscle group, and the use of free weights or machines. The number of possible programs was 10 to the sixty-seventh power. "That's why a magazine can come up with a new program every day and, Kraemer says, a company can always brag, 'We've got the new program.' "

ten

THE FITNESS BUSINESS

I'm using the shoulder-press machine in the weight room of the New York Sports Club near my office and watching my friend Erica as she wanders over to a machine that exercises the trapezius muscles. She stares at it, wondering how to use it. You should ask one of the trainers when you can't figure out a machine, I tell her. It has never occurred to her. "Don't you have to pay?" she wonders.

It does seem that there are two kinds of people at the gym—those who move from exercise to exercise on their own and those who pay for sessions with a personal trainer and then spend their time at the gym trailing this person around the weight-room floor, getting help and instruction with each machine and each exercise that requires dumbbells or barbells. Or they go to the machines like treadmills and elliptical trainers, allowing their trainers to push the buttons on the machines, setting them for ten or twenty minutes of exercise. People like Erica, who have no experience lifting, fumble on alone, feeling like outsiders, intimidated by many of the machines.

And I understand why she never thought to ask for help; the trainers do look preoccupied. I know they are well aware of how to lift weights because I have seen some of them at their own workouts before their shifts begin. But what they do with clients often is very different.

There is Gabe, a slender young man with high cheekbones and short black hair; he's training a plump woman wearing black tights, white sneakers, and a long white T-shirt. He asks her to stand against a wall and hold her right leg straight out in front of her. Slowly, gradually, he pulls it upward, stretching her hamstring.

Across the room, another trainer is working with a middle-aged man whose body has grown soft. She has her client lying on his back on a narrow bench, a fifteen-pound weight in each hand. Slowly, he raises his arms and brings the weights together above his chest, while she stands behind the bench, guiding his arms, aiding him in lifting.

It all seems very gentle and nonthreatening. I almost expect to hear New Age music in the background. And since these trainers are certified professionals, I might well assume that whatever they are doing is going to make a difference in their clients' muscle development or flexibility or weight.

I first learned about the qualifications of fitness trainers when my daughter, Therese, decided to get certified. I thought it would be an arduous task. Larry Gambrell, who taught me to lift weights, was not certified—he was afraid to take the test even though he seemed to know a lot about how to lift and how to design an exercise program. Somehow, I had this notion that a certified personal trainer was like a board-certified orthodontist. To be certified, orthodontists have to show how they took ten clients— their teeth protruding or overlapping or caving in—from an initial visit, to a plan of action, its implementation, and finally to the point where their teeth are lined up correctly. You can be an orthodontist without being board certified: any dentist can simply declare himself to be an orthodontist, but board certification provides evidence that they should be able to produce the results they are promising.

Personal trainers, I used to think, must be required to create a fitness plan for a few typical clients, people who were out of shape, with little or no muscle tone, perhaps no endurance, not sure which muscle is their triceps and which their quadriceps. The qualifying trainers would be able to show that after working with these clients, they had helped them to remake their bodies.

Was I wrong.

It was the end of the summer of 2001 and Therese had just resigned from an intense job in investment banking that was requiring her to travel back and forth from Bangkok once or twice a month and live most of the time in hotels. She needed a break and thought it would be fun to work in a gym. Since she knew how to lift, she decided to become a personal trainer. She asked around at a few gyms and learned that if she were certified by the American Council on Exercise, or ACE, most gyms would hire her. It's an organization that began in 1985 and claims to have certified more than 45,000 people since then, in the United States and seventy-seven other countries. It offers several types of certification—personal trainer, group fitness instructor, lifestyle and weight management consultant, clinical exercise specialist. Therese signed up to become an ACE-certified personal trainer.

It turned out to be easy—all she had to do was take and pass a written exam. She did not have to show she knew her way around a weight room or that she knew how to run or how to use an elliptical trainer. She did not have to see a single client, nor did she even have to set foot in a gym. But she did have to pay. She had a choice, either sign up for a $299 exam preparation course or buy a home-study guide for $295. Then she had to pay $200 to take the exam. She chose the home-study guide, paying by phone with a credit card.

A huge package arrived in the mail, containing a heavy textbook, a 160-page study guide, flashcards, six audio cassettes, a schedule for studying and reviewing all the chapters in the book, a practice exam, and the Internet address for a site with online review questions. Therese glanced through the book, expecting to learn what exercises a trainer can use to help a client develop specific muscle groups. But that, it turned out, was not what the book was about. Rather, most of the book focused on how to assess a client's fitness level, how to deal with their medical problems, emphasizing repeatedly that trainers are not doctors and should not try to give medical advice. Most importantly, the book stressed how to encourage clients to sign up for more personal training sessions. What about how to use the health club's machines and weights? "Maybe they thought that was something you would learn on the job," Therese says.

She studied for a few days prior to taking the exam, and then she took the practice test, which revealed that she did not know much about human anatomy. So she tried to quickly memorize all the muscles of the body and their functions. The exam was the next day and Therese began to worry. One problem was that she was still uncertain about how well she had to do. The ACE Web site did not reveal what a passing score was. It said only: "The total number of correct answers determines your raw score, which is then scaled statistically to ensure that all versions of the exam are equal in difficulty and content." All you need to do is pass—it's not like college, where a grade-point average matters—but it was impossible to tell from taking the practice tests how many answers you needed to get right.

Therese arrived at an office building in Manhattan on a Saturday morning and looked around at the forty or so people there. Few of them, she thought, looked like they had spent much time in a gym. Or, if they had, they had not benefited from it. Most, she says, "were people who looked like they were semi-in-shape, who may have been high school athletes. Many of them had little muscle tone, and although none were fat, they just looked like the typical people you might see in a gym, not really in shape but not really out of shape, either." While most of the people were in their twenties and thirties, there was one man and one woman who were at least sixty, Therese guessed.

The exam itself was a surprise. It was a typical multiple-choice test with 175 questions that students answered by filling in bubbles beside their answers with number-two pencils. Little was asked about human anatomy. Instead, a typical question asked what one should do to motivate a tired client.

"I left the exam thinking I was sure I had passed," Therese recalls. After all, she was always a good student, the sort who effortlessly gets high scores on standardized tests, and she had a bachelor's degree in economics from the University of Pennsylvania. How hard could it be to pass a personal-trainer exam? But then she began to feel a sort of nagging anxiety. Who knew what were the right answers to such vague questions? And what was a passing score?

Her results came in the mail a couple of weeks later. She passed.

Within two weeks, having never trained anyone in her life, she was working at a New Jersey health club. She did have to go through a brief apprenticeship, however, following trainers around for two weeks before taking on clients of her own. The gym charged clients $64 for a single session or $540 for a package of ten. Therese's fee was always the same, $23 for each hour-long session she booked.

So, after five days of perfunctory study, a multiple-choice exam that focused on the business of getting and keeping clients, an outlay of $495, and a short training period at her health club, Therese was working as a certified personal trainer.

Soon, Therese decided she would like to get another certification, as a Spinning instructor. Her gym would pay her $22 for each Spinning class she taught and, like me, she loves to spin. So she went to the Spinning Web site and began the process of becoming certified.

Anyone can also be a certified Spinning instructor. You do not have to be strong or fit. You do not have to know anything about Spinning—you can do it without ever having previously set foot in a Spinning class. It takes one day. And it costs $275, plus

$29.95 for an instructor's manual. This time, the certification process took place in a Philadelphia gym. Therese arrived at nine a.m., with everything she had been told to bring—two sets of gym clothes to wear during two Spinning classes, food for lunch, a water bottle, a notebook, and a pen.

It was a nine-hour day, and the students never left the Spinning room.

The instructor, or presenter, as they are called, was Lisa Sherman Dow, a tall athletic woman with short brown hair and freckles. She was slim and strong, with long legs that were slender and muscular—like the legs of the teenagers Larry was training the night that sold me on weight lifting—and she had the fluid movements of a natural athlete. But the other people in the class did not look nearly so fit.

Of the dozen or so people in the class besides Therese, about eight were nearing middle age and were out of shape and pudgy. Only one of them looked truly athletic.

"After we had introduced ourselves, we got down to business," Therese says. "We were given our Johnny G Spinning manuals and we were told we were going to learn how to set up the bike," getting instructions on how to arrange the level of the seat and its distance from the handlebars and how high to slide the handlebars. They then began a Spinning class. Lisa showed them how to ride in the approved positions while sitting and standing on the bikes.

"Of course, the room was full of mirrors, so I made sure to look at everyone," Therese admitted. "Most of the people seemed as though they were having trouble learning how to ride correctly, especially during the standing portions"—when you grasp the handlebars but do not put most of your weight on your hands. "Lisa tried to correct these mistakes but I really don't think they all walked out of there with perfect technique."

Then it was time for lunch, followed by a lecture on the Johnny G "Energy Zones," the different classes that are supposed to emphasize endurance, strength, interval training, or a fast-paced class called Race Day. They learned to use Johnny G symbols to plan their class. To denote a seated climb, which entails sitting on the bike with the resistance on the pedals high enough so it feels like you are climbing a hill, you darken the bottom half of a square. For a standing climb, you darken the top half of the box.

As you move through the manual, the symbols become more and more complicated. There are symbols for cadence checks, for resistance loading (which means staying at the same pace and increasing your resistance), and for heart-rate checks.

The day ended with another Spinning session, the group riding for fifteen minutes in each energy zone. And then the class was dismissed. Therese and her class were certified Johnny G Spinning instructors.

I understand, of course, the need for certification—those who design programs like Spinning want to be sure that classes with their name are conducted as they intended. At least one organization, the American College of Sports Medicine, takes certification seriously. Its "health and fitness instructor" certification, for example, requires that the person major in a field like exercise science at an accredited college or university or have nine hundred hours of practical experience. The group holds workshops lasting several days for certification candidates. Its test requires that the candidates pass a written exam and a sixty-minute practical exam, in which they must demonstrate an ability to assess a client's fitness and develop an exercise program.

But, for the most part, certification is a business. ACE and Mad Dogg Athletics, which owns the Spinning trademark, and virtually every other group that gives certifications for personal training or for teaching special classes, do not just ask those it certifies to pay once. Instead, they require that you pay for continuing education credits each year to remain certified.

My favorite is the take-home multiple-choice quizzes that the

organizations send their certified instructors. For a small pay-
ment, you can get points to keep your certification current.
Johnny G, for example, sends out newsletters with a quiz at the
end consisting of true-false questions. Every question is explicitly
answered in the newsletter. But some of the answers are pretty
obvious. True or false, one question asked, "Fatigue is not a goal
during warm-up." You send in your answers along with $20. If
you get thirteen out of fifteen right answers, you get a bonus
point. You need to send in certificates showing you earned fourteen points in two years, along with a processing fee of $69.95 to
stay certified.

ACE does the same thing, but it only requires that you get six
out of ten correct answers in its take-home multiple-choice test.
You circle your answers, send in $10, and if you pass you get 0.1
continuing-education credits toward the 1.5 you need each year.
And just in case you have trouble with the questions, you can
turn the page upside down and see the answers.

Of course, other, more expensive programs can get you more
credits. ACE offers an "Exercise for Older Adults Correspon-
dence Study Course" for $69. You get a manual, a video, and a
quiz. Send in your answers to the quiz questions with a $10 pro-
cessing fee and, if you pass, you get 0.5 ACE points. Mad Dogg
Athletics has a home-study course called "Periodization for Peak
Performance" that costs $79.95 but gives you 4 Spinning points
and 0.4 ACE points.

Both groups have conventions, with opportunities to earn still
more points. At the December–January 2002 Spinning convention in Miami, participants could sign up for a Mount Everest
ride with Josh Taylor. It was held the day before the convention
began, costing $75 and earning participants 3 Spinning points.
Unlike the group at Evolutions Fitness, the convention participants did not train for weeks beforehand. And the ride was an
hour shorter.

The conventions are not cheap. Instructors paid $399 to regis-
ter for the August 2002 Spinning meeting in Chicago. For an ex-

tra $99, they could spend the day before the meeting exercising with Johnny G. Or they could spend four hours before the meeting getting certified as a YogaButt instructor, described as "an exciting new program that targets the thighs, gluteals, and abdominals." It costs $69 to get this certification, but it comes with 0.4 ACE points and 2 Spinning points.

At the meeting itself, you could go to an hour-long lecture on the "Anatomy of a Pedal Stroke" or one titled "Delicate Devouring: Getting the Most from Your Food Choices." You could take a workshop called "It's a Pain: Dealing with Discomfort." Or, if you are a Spinning program director, you might want to go to a session called "How to Turn Your Spinning Program into a New Profit Center."

One company, ECA World Fitness, specializes in continuing education and conventions. At its meeting in Miami in November of 2002, it offered continuing-education credits not just for Spinning and ACE but for ten other groups as well. It also offered certification to teach trademarked classes, like Fittrek, described as "an innovative and progressive program that is teaching members and instructors to think out of the box!" It costs $199 for ECA members and $209 for nonmembers to be certified, but you get continuing-education points for ACE as well as for another group, AFAA.

Then there are the products, and not just logo items like the Spinning bike jerseys for $48.75 or the shorts for $54.95 or the Spinning bandannas for $6.95 each. There are also books, tapes, equipment, special foods, drinks, and supplements that are marketed to trainers. There is even a company, Exercise, Etc., that is like the *Princeton Review* of the trainer certification industry. It offers exam prep courses and home-study courses and continuing-education courses.

The parade of new programs is never-ending. Gyms in my area, including Gold's and Evolutions, began offering a new trademarked program called Body Pump. It is a tightly choreographed group class of weight lifting to music. Phyllis Zenda, the group fitness director at the Gold's Gym where I am a member, told me she was sold on the program when she saw a Body Pump presenter who was stunningly fit and handsome and who told his audience that Body Pump was the only exercise he did.

Is there any evidence that it works, I wonder? Body Pump classes are still in session on Wednesday nights when our Spinning class has just ended, and I often stare through the glass walls at the Body Pumpers while I wait for Bill to change out of his sweaty clothes. They seem to be doing endless repetitions with relatively low weights—not a prescription for building muscles. The reason to believe it works, of course, is that the company that sells it says it does. But there is one study, published in 2000 in the *Journal of Strength and Conditioning Research* by investigators at the University of Texas at Austin. They monitored fifteen men and fifteen women during a Body Pump workout. Their conclusion? "Responses were below that necessary to elicit an aerobic-training effect and were lower than responses previously reported with circuit weight training."

Six months after the start of Body Pump, Gold's Gym launched its successor, Body Attack. The gym had a countdown to the first class, crossing off the days remaining until Memorial Day 2002, when its members could experience for themselves this new combination of Tae Bo–type movements (a fast-paced combination of martial arts punching and jabbing and aerobics) with lifting. And, of course, the Body Attack instructors are certified by the developers of the program.

Unlike the pharmaceutical industry, which is regulated by the Food and Drug Administration and cannot make unsubstantiated claims, and unlike academia, where scientists maintain their credibility by publishing papers in peer-reviewed journals, the fitness business has few bounds.

Publicists pepper reporters with e-mails.

"Hi," writes Jessica Berger of MCR Communications in an

e-mail whose subject is "INTERVIEW WITH YANKEES TRAIN-ING COACH." I've never heard of her, but the breezy greeting is de rigueur. "I thought if you were writing anything about fitness devices or sports rehabilitation it might pique your interest to find out how the athletes train and prevent injuries for their big events. One of the most instrumental prepatory [sic] training and rehabilitation devices that is used by many of the participants is a fitness tool called the Bodyblade. This workout tool has made tremendous strides in the athletic industry over the years, and re-cently in the consumer market.

"The Bodyblade is the quintessential device in the training rooms for just about every pro-sport team in the nation, including The Yankees, The Patriots, The Diamondbacks, The Chicago Bulls, The Dolphins, et al.

"A new study, which has been released in the January 2002 is-sue of the *Journal of Orthopedic Sports Physical Therapy* re-vealed that (in conjunction with a daily fitness regimen) the Bodyblade improves sports performance significantly and PRE-VENTS injury.

"This will not come as a shock to strength and conditioning coaches, like Gene Monohan of the NY Yankees, who swears by it, saying that players who he regularly uses it with have im-proved their strength, agility, posture and balance coordination." She adds that the device also helped players recover from injuries, especially to their shoulders and spines. "Gene also trains with the blade for core stabilization—including abs, trunks, and flanks," she writes.

"In the consumer market, expect to see Bodyblade in health clubs across the country and sold as retail as well as utilized in fit-ness classes. There are different size variations of the blade, so men, women and children can choose one that suits their needs. Smaller blades for cardiovascular; larger blades for strength train-ing. Prices range from $49–$204."

She concludes by offering me an interview with Monohan of the Yankees, but never tells me what the blade is. I check its Web site, which has a lot of pseudoscientific babble about Newton's laws of motion and pictures of people who seem to be waving a flexible rod in front of them. That rod is the blade.

Perhaps I should not be so cynical. Time after time, I see programs that gain adherents despite a glaring lack of evidence that they are any better than the routines they are meant to replace. SuperSlow, for example, is a special program whose main feature is a slow-motion lifting and lowering of weights that has inspired some people to lift their weights more slowly than ever, whether or not they are following the official program. Its inventor, Ken Hutchins, says he invented it when he was working as a trainer for a study at the University of Florida Medical School on weight training in elderly women. Hutchins had previously competed in powerlifting and was working for Nautilus, which sponsored the study. He says the study researchers reported that the women did not improve with the program, but he knows better. "So what does this tell you about all those silly tests they make you take at the local wellness center?" he asks. Hutchins left Nautilus in 1988 to introduce his SuperSlow program to the nation's exercisers.

The ACE magazine for personal trainers made SuperSlow its cover story for the March–April 2002 issue but, to its credit, the organization at least injected a note of skepticism in its article, titled "Superslow: One Man's Defiant Challenge."

The idea is to do one set of five or six exercises to failure, raising or lowering weights very slowly, taking ten seconds to raise a weight and another ten to lower it. Also, to do it right, you are supposed to lift and lower these weights in a room that is cool and dry with no mirrors, music, or any other distractions. You are to be guided by certified SuperSlow trainers. And the promise is that if you do this program just once or twice a week, your muscles will grow big and strong and, as an added bonus, you will get all the cardiovascular benefits of aerobic exercise.

One group at George Washington University Medical Center tested the program in women, publishing its findings in 2001 in the *Journal of Strength and Conditioning Research*. The investigators trained women three times a week, one group with a traditional weight-lifting program, the other with SuperSlow. They found that the traditional program was better for building muscle strength and that the SuperSlow program, Hutchins's claims to the contrary, did not improve the women's ability to do sustained active exercise the way a program such as running would.

Hutchins told the ACE magazine that he does not need research to prove his claims. "I don't like quoting research papers, because most of the studies are so poorly performed that they aren't worth it."

In a sense, I can't entirely disagree. But while the George Washington University study had only fourteen subjects, half of them did serve as a comparison group, which is essential if one is to assess a program's effects. And it did draw on extensive knowledge of what would be expected if a program worked. It seems to me that the onus should be on Hutchins and that a failure to find statistically significant evidence that a program works is not to be dismissed. But in general, it is an unfortunate fact of exercise life that those who are selling the products and programs end up as the sole authorities on their effectiveness.

Hutchins is hardly reticent about claiming benefits for SuperSlow. Not only does the program help healthy people get in shape, he says, but he also has used it to successfully treat patients with Parkinson's disease, spinal fusion, urinary incontinence, and sexual dysfunction.

Of course, there is a certification process, through the SuperSlow Exercise Guild. I check the Web site and learn that you start by mailing in your application, with a $595 fee. Then you buy the instructional books and videos and arrange to be tested. If you want to go on and become an advanced, Level II, SuperSlow instructor, it will cost you another $795.

Hutchins does not try to make his test easy. He describes one part of a practical exam, which accompanies the written test for Level II aspirants: "The neck part of the practical lasts 2–3 hours. Exercise for the neck is a tedious undertaking involving a delicate area of the body that the rest of the fitness industry avoids and should avoid, because they do not know what they are doing, and because what they practice and promote as exercise is going to maim and kill people if they apply their nonsense to the neck. The application of specialized neck information enables me to personally evaluate the examinee, not just related to neck exercise, but it also enables me to gain a perspective on the examinee's competence and get in sync with the Master who certified him Level-I. In addition, the examinee is expected to keep my hours and follow me as an intern with my clients throughout the week.

"Assuming that he completes the Level-II, and assuming that I trust him to properly represent the Guild and SuperSlow, the examinee is given the option to be appointed a Master. As a Master he is then an officer in the Guild and has the authority to administer Level-I Certifications. To maintain this status it is expected that he will attend the National Guild Convention each year."

No one has yet failed the Level II test, Hutchins writes, adding, however, that he has discouraged some from taking it.

While the ACE magazine article does quote some skeptics, it also cites enthusiasts and tells trainers how to do the routine, complete with large color photographs demonstrating the five basic exercises. It adds a caveat: "While Hutchins claims his protocol can only be administered by a trainer certified by him (or, if that's not possible, by ordering training videotapes from Hutchins's Web site) some experts believe it is possible to do a SuperSlow workout on your own."

I know—SuperSlow is a marginal program. While it may have a few adherents plus a few who went on to become Level II instructors (successfully completing even the neck exam), compared to something like Spinning, it has never really caught on. Most gyms have Spinning classes. Very few have SuperSlow programs. Maybe success or failure depends on the zeal of the program's founder.

Johnny G got his program into health clubs through unflagging persistence. He and his partner traveled all over the country, lugging the heavy Spinning bike from gym to gym, trying for four years to persuade club owners to offer their program. Finally, Schwinn licensed the bike and began producing and marketing it. They named it the Johnny G Spinner and introduced it at the 1995 convention of the International Health, Racquet & Sportsclub Association, the major health-club trade group. "That was the turning point," Johnny wrote.

I asked him if those days are over now that Spinning is established. Not at all, he said. He never lets up. When I spoke to him in July of 2002, he had just returned from three months of international travel. After five days at home, he would be off again for another three months, selling his program. In the past few years, he said, he has traveled over a million miles.

"The stationary bike has always been perceived as the most boring piece of equipment in the world. You have to show it live," Johnny explains. So he goes to conventions and trade shows and he puts on special Spinning events with hundreds of people riding Spinning bikes for hours.

Special programs like Spinning are, of course, only a tiny slice of the exercise business. There are more than 17,000 health clubs in America today. One out of every eight adult Americans is a member; the total number of members is 32.8 million. The median amount of money coming into a health club in 2002 was $5,116,000. And these clubs are just a fragment of the exercise business that has grown up in my adult lifetime.

I look at my collection of running shoes—one pair to wear when I run outdoors and two old pairs to wear at the gym. From the days when I started running, in tennis shoes, until now, an entire industry and mystique has built up around shoes alone. The National Sporting Goods Association reports that in 2001 the sales of footwear for sports reached $13.3 billion.

Of course, not everyone is convinced that the claims of shoe manufacturers hold up to scientific scrutiny. At a recent conference in England, one expert, Trevor Prior of St. Leonard's

Primary Care Center in London, noted that "many shoe manufacturers are purporting to have specific technology incorporated into their shoes to either control pronation or facilitate function, depending on foot type and activity level. It is difficult to obtain scientific data relating to these injuries."

He cites as an example claims that shoes cushion shock. "It is easy to demonstrate the basic rearfoot control provided by different shoes with simple video technology," Prior said. But, he added, at least one research study has suggested that cushioned shoes can give the runner an illusion that the impact of the feet on the ground is less than it really is, thus "predisposing to injury," Prior noted.

Shoe manufacturers use video cameras and special force measurements to design and test their shoes. "Although much data is available from these studies, a clear picture of normal and abnormal function has yet to be developed," says Prior. And that lack of understanding is compounded when orthopedists and podiatrists attempt to treat and prevent injuries by prescribing special inserts, known as orthotics, to go inside of shoes.

Another participant at the conference, Martyn Shorten, a managing partner of Biomechanica, a company in Oregon, said much the same. One obsessive focus of shoe manufacturers and doctors attempting to prevent injuries is so-called pronation control, an attempt to ease excessive inward rotation of the foot and lower leg when the foot hits the ground. "Detailed mechanism of injury and treatment through pronation control, however, are still not well understood," notes Shorten. As for shoe inserts that reduce the motion at the rear of the foot, at least one study found no difference in foot motion when runners used any of six different inserts as compared to when they used no inserts.

Food, of course, is another major obsession of the exercise field. There are the special diets and supplements promoted by health clubs. At Gold's Gym, the program is called Apex, and it has its own Apex Certified Fitness Professionals (gym employees who went on to get Apex certification) who will help you reach your goals, the company claims. The program, which combines supplements with personal training, quotes glowing testimonials from satisfied clients with identifiers like "T.C., Wisconsin" and "J.S., California," and even has held nationwide contests for the best before-and-after photos.

Luxury health clubs that are run by The Sports Club/LA in Los Angeles, New York, and Washington, D.C., have their own program, the PTS, or Personal Trainer System, which includes a diet, an exercise program, and nutritional supplements prescribed by a certified employee. The company touts its results in a press release: "Member 'Judy Whitledge' lost nine and a half pounds in just four weeks and gained one pound of muscle." And, the press release adds, member Anne Behringer says, "I feel incredible! My energy levels are way up without peaks or valleys throughout the day. I feel stronger than ever; the 45 pound bench press bar seems light. I feel much leaner and I've lost my appetite for junk food."

Then there is the exploding industry that sells hope and promises of weight loss and muscle definition and strength and endurance through food and food supplements. *Men's Fitness* seems to devote half of its pages to advertisements for these products. In the March 2002 issue there is the full-page ad for the "delicious meal replacement food bar," that promises to "support lean muscle," another full-page ad for a sports drink that says it will "jolt your metabolism" with the "fat-burning stack of Ma Huang," as well as caffeine, white willow bark, quercetin, L-carnetine, and niacin. The ad does not mention that the Food and Drug Administration has warned that healthy people have reported suffering a variety of ill effects from Ma Huang, ranging from episodes of high blood pressure, irregular heart rates, and tremors, to seizures, strokes, and death. Adding caffeine makes matters even worse.

Still another full-page ad in that issue hawks a diet pill just for men that is "unmatched in its ability to attack stubborn abdominal fat deposits." Then there is the three-page advertisement for "slow-release protein complexes that you drink at night, right before you go to bed" that are supposed to help you grow muscles while you sleep.

Just in case you'd rather not ingest anything, the same issue has a full-page advertisement for a "Ripping Gel," which promises that all you have to do is massage it into your skin over your abdomen and it will penetrate and melt fat away. The prices can be hefty. A 3.78-ounce, one-month supply of Ripping Gel will set you back $109; the men-only diet pills run $59 for a one-month supply.

Most scientists just roll their eyes when I ask them about these products. Many recite the old P. T. Barnum line about a sucker being born every minute. Larry Rome, however, the muscle researcher at the University of Pennsylvania, takes a stab at answering questions about one of the chemicals that is marketed to exercisers.

Rome fields practical questions about supplements often because some of the men who work at a delicatessen he frequents are bodybuilders, and they ask him if they should take creatine supplements. Does it really build muscle?

He tells them to save their money. The supplements can't make them stronger, and he explains why. To give the substance the benefit of the doubt, he will assume that it is physiologically active, that it is carried by the blood to the muscles, which take it up in appropriate doses, increasing the body's natural supply of creatine. But, he asks, then what? What is the consequence?

If you call on your muscles for a powerful burst of energy, the sort of demand a sprinter might make on his thigh muscles, the most immediate fuel supply is adenosine triphosphate, or ATP, a molecule that is split to release energy to cells. However, your muscles would use up their entire ATP supply in a second or two, at which point the muscle would go into rigor and become stiff. This, in fact, is what happens after death, in rigor mortis, when muscles use up their ATP and become rigid. But living muscle, Rome explains, has a protective mechanism that replenishes ATP as fast as it is being broken down until the muscles can gear up their enzymes to provide energy from the glycogen in the muscles. The compound that is responsible for this rapid replenishment of ATP is called creatine phosphate.

In other words: the muscles call on an energy source, ATP, for an immediate blast of fuel. They use their stored ATP for a few seconds, until their enzymes can begin producing energy from glycogen. And if the muscles run out of ATP before new energy is available to them from glycogen, they break down stored creatine, in the form of creatine phosphate, to make more ATP.

The problem, Rome says, is that although there is about five times as much creatine phosphate as ATP in muscles, its supply is still limited. That led to the notion that if you ingest creatine supplements you can build muscles. Of course, it makes no scientific sense.

"Creatine phosphate provides power for five to ten seconds if you are doing a hundred-yard sprint," says Rome. But if you are lifting weights, "the only advantage it could possibly give you is if you are doing very rapid repetitions. Maybe it could give you the ability to do one more rep. In an hour of constant exercise, it would only help you in the first few seconds."

Rome can speculate about why some weight lifters swear by it. When you take massive doses of creatine, your muscles absorb water along with it. "More water goes in, the muscle looks bigger, and people say, 'Oh man, that stuff is great.'" But they have no more muscle protein. Their muscles are no stronger, and the extra water will leak out again.

With all these companies and all these products competing in the same market, I wonder how any succeed. Why would anyone buy the Ripping Gel as opposed to the supplements called "Animal Cuts"? Or why use either of these when you can get human growth hormone, advertised in *Men's Fitness*. It is a prescription drug, and most doctors would refuse to prescribe it for healthy people. But the ad, in the March 2002 issue, tells you how to get a prescription: "Call for a list of physicians near you." The ad promises that human growth hormone will not only increase your muscle mass but get rid of fat, reverse aging, strengthen the immune system, improve sexual performance, and lower blood pressure and cholesterol. It fails to mention that the Food and Drug Administration has approved growth hormone only for the treatment of children with kidney disease and children and adults with genetic defects that prevent them from making the hormone. As evidence that growth hormone could increase muscle mass in adults ads often cite a small study of twenty-one elderly men published in 1990 in the *New England Journal of Medicine*. Other claims have not been established, and the small study showing muscle gain falls far short of the sort of evidence that would be required by the FDA if a company wanted to market the drug for such a use. In fact, the results of a subsequent larger study, published in the *Annals of Internal Medicine* in 1996, were far less rosy. It involved fifty-two elderly men, half of whom got a placebo, and found that those who took it got no stronger and suffered side effects such as puffy ankles and aching joints.

And why would Bodyblade be able to employ a marketing firm and sell its flexible rod? How did SuperSlow ever gain a following, even meriting a spot on a National Public Radio program? Who dreams up programs like YogaButt? And who, I ask, would really want to try something like Irving Dardik's Heart Waves program? Who are all these people who seem to be so willing to spend so much money on products, programs, and devices that have nothing but marketing and promotion behind them?

I get a call from Kathryn Schwartz about another special Spinning ride that will be held at Evolutions Fitness. It will be led by Josh Taylor and his friend Bill Perrault, but it will be very different from Mount Everest. This time, we will train for a ride to simulate part of a one-day, 180-mile race that takes place each year in Italy. It's known as the Giro d'Italia, and it has a reputation for being one of the toughest races in bicycling. We'll ride for just three hours, pretending we are covering the section from Milan to San Remo. Instead of training for endurance, like we did with Mount Everest, we will be training for sprints, strength, and speed. To whet our appetites, we can come to Evolutions for a ninety-minute ride with Josh on Friday night. Are we interested? Of course.

Bill and I arrive about fifteen minutes early for the Friday night ride. A Body Pump class is in session in the exercise room at Evolutions, so we wait quietly outside the room, watching the group do their final exercises, abdominal crunches.

A chunky middle-aged man comes up to me. I recognize him immediately from the Mount Everest ride. It's Arnold. He still looks the same.

Arnold remembers me, too, and he has some news for me. He was so elated when he finished the Mount Everest ride that he got certified as a Spinning instructor and is now teaching classes six mornings a week, at three gyms. And, he adds, he just met the most amazing man on an airplane. He was an executive with a company that had invented an exciting and revolutionary form of exercise that Arnold predicted could sweep the country.

And what, I ask, is this program called?

"Heart Waves," says Arnold.

THE TRUTH ABOUT EXERCISE

I don't give health advice, I like to tell anyone who asks. I'm a reporter, not a doctor, not a scientist. My job is just to give you the information that might allow you to think for yourself. If there's one group that annoys me it's the self-appointed people who act like health police, who shake their heads in dismay at those who do not eat or exercise just as they do, and who explain in all earnestness that they are protecting themselves from cancer by eating blueberries or tomatoes or that they are full of energy because they walk a mile each morning. I once met a retired police officer while reporting for the *New York Times* who asked me to feel his bicep. Proof, he said, that he was healthy, that he took care of himself, unlike those fat and sloppy masses out there.

But maybe the fitness arena is different from medicine, my usual focus. Now that I have come to appreciate the sketchiness of fitness science and the breadth of fitness marketing, I have a few answers for people who ask me: "What should I do to get fit?"

If I learned anything from investigating the exercise field, it is that good research often gets lost amidst marketing claims and exaggerations and the sale of dubious programs and nostrums. Yet there is valid research that can be trusted. This is research conducted not for marketing purposes but for the purposes of scientific inquiry. It involves studies that include control groups and that look for results that are statistically significant, that are highly unlikely to have occurred by chance. It tends to be done by academic researchers who want to learn the truth, not to prove a pet hypothesis (or a commercially driven hypothesis). That means that they are as willing to say that a hoped-for benefit did not emerge as that it did.

So if someone wants to start exercising, I would suggest paying attention to studies that have these hallmarks of validity. And then I would ask: What are you trying to accomplish? And why? There seem to be three principal reasons for exercising, and what is needed for one goal is not necessarily what is needed for another.

If your goal is to improve your health, studies in recent years have consistently indicated that you get the most benefit when you go from no exercise at all to exercising moderately. Starting with Steve Blair's classic study "Physical Fitness and All-Cause Mortality" (1989), a convincing body of research has emerged in support of the observation that most of the health benefit probably occurs from just mild exercise, not necessarily from the most arduous workouts.

The good news is that what the researchers call moderate exercise really is moderate. Most health benefits seem to accrue if you simply walk briskly for about 20 to 30 minutes a day, covering a mile in 15 to 20 minutes, or ride a bike at a modest pace. You can take three 10-minute walks a day, or you can ride a bike for 20 minutes and walk for 10. Or you can swim at a comfortable pace for all or part of your exercise program. Almost any physical activity will suffice, and there is no need to push yourself till you're out of breath, gasping for air. You don't have to return from your session soaked in sweat. Yes, you do get a slight extra benefit from exercising a little harder or a little longer, but that extra benefit is small compared to the benefit you apparently get from just doing moderate exercise.

As Michael Lauer, the Cleveland Clinic cardiologist, tells me, "Riding a bike can be a lot of fun, but you might think that the only way to get a cardiovascular benefit would be to ride for thirty miles a day. The point is—no, that's not correct. You can take a thirty-minute easy bike ride and still get a real cardiovascular benefit. What we are asking for," he clarified, "are very mild levels of activity, but they need to occur pretty often."

When it comes to the benefits of strength training, the extensive body of evidence in the position paper written by the American College of Sports Medicine documents that it can improve muscle strength, make everyday life easier, and prevent falls. Decades of research by exercise physiologists show that resistance exercise can change the muscle cells in positive ways. As Claude Bouchard, for example, confirmed in his large study of inherited differences in the ability to train, muscle that is developed with exercise is more efficient, has more mitochondria, and is better at using fat for fuel and at allowing cells to use insulin to utilize blood sugar, thus making diabetes less likely.

But it is not easy to walk into a weight room at a gym and just start lifting.

For advice on how to do it, I defer to William Kraemer, one of the leading experts on strength training, editor of a scientific journal on the subject, and lead author of the position statement on strength training by the American College of Sports Medicine. I asked him if novices would do well to read books or magazines like *Shape*, or *Men's Health*, or *Muscle & Fitness*.

"Not an easy answer—maybe all of them, if they can get accurate information and not become a victim to infomercial hype and inaccurate information," Kraemer replied. "It's a jungle out there, and each individual has different needs, so start with an organization like the National Strength and Conditioning Association" (a nonprofit professional group with headquarters in Colorado Springs and a Web site, nsca-lift.org). "Do not be afraid to challenge yourself and *think*," he insists. "Information should be evaluated and its source should be known."

But I also think that the health benefits of exercise can be oversold. They probably are real, but they are not necessarily dramatic.

Will you as an individual live longer if you exercise? That's not clear. There appears to be an effect in an entire population, but it takes large numbers of people to show it. For example, Blair's study involved more than 13,000 healthy men and women who were followed for eight years. During that time, 283 died. The investigators used statistical models to calculate how likely it was that a person would die in a given year. In the lowest fitness category for men, 75 out of 14,515 would die, as compared to 35 out of 17,557 in the highest fitness category. For women, 18 out of every 4,916 in the lowest fitness category would be expected to die in a year, compared to 4 out of every 4,613 who were most fit.

Even that effect has a question mark over it. Blair's study, like every study of exercise and health, has a fundamental flaw—it observes people who happen to exercise, or happen not to exercise, and asks how healthy they are. Researchers use statistics to correct for differences between the groups because, as might be expected, those who exercise tend to be healthier to start with than those who do not. Such statistical adjustments can only go so far, however, because scientists can never be assured that they have accounted for all the differences.

The problem of statistical corrections is a well-known pitfall of observational studies, and one that has tripped up scientists on other important questions, such as the benefits of hormone replacement therapy in postmenopausal women. Women in the observational studies were healthier when they took estrogen and progestin. It turned out, however, that healthy women were the ones taking hormones; it was not the hormones that made them healthy. In fact, hormone therapy turned out to have slight health risks, making it inadvisable for most women to take it for long periods of time.

The ideal way to do an exercise study, and the way that the hormone replacement question finally was answered, is to randomly assign one group of people to undergo a treatment (in this case, hormones) and another group to forgo the intervention, and then wait to see who has better health. Such a study of exercise will never be done. No one knows how they could get people in one group to agree to exercise regularly for years and equal numbers in another group to agree to be sedentary. Even if they could, the study would require huge numbers of people to see an effect, because exercise, at best, creates relatively small changes in a population's health. It simply is infeasible. For the foreseeable future, there is no choice but to accept, or dismiss, the large observational studies. I accept them, while realizing their limitations. If the studies have come to the wrong conclusion, all that would mean is that an imagined small benefit of exercise may in fact be nonexistent.

When it comes to the health benefits of weight lifting, most are not based on solid evidence. For example, physiologists say it is not true that weight lifting will raise your metabolic rate, and osteoporosis experts say there is no rigorous study showing it will reduce your risk of osteoporosis.

The second reason to exercise is to improve your appearance and your performance. You may want to be thinner, or stronger. In this case, moderate exercise is unlikely to be enough. Whether you lose weight may depend on how hard you exercise, how long, what you eat, and what your genetics are. Obesity experts often say you can just walk—a half-hour or so of brisk walking will burn maybe 150 calories. In a month, if you do not change your diet, you could lose a pound. It really is much more effective to exercise hard enough to sweat, and that is the only way to burn large numbers of calories.

Whether you grow stronger or reshape your body depends on a lot of factors, including your genes, but also including how often you lift weights, whether the weights are heavy enough to stress your muscles, and whether you stay with your program.

The exercise that will make you thinner and more muscular, the sort that will allow you to run faster or swim for longer distances, requires not just consistency but effort. Or, as exercise physiologist Donald Kirkendall says: "If you want to push performance, you've got to push the intensity. The biggest way to gain fitness is to push intensity."

The third reason for exercise is almost never the impetus for starting. Instead, it is one that tends to creep up on people, taking them by surprise. Yet it is the one that often accounts for them staying with an exercise program. Time and again, when I ask people why they keep exercising, year in and year out, they tell me that they started exercising to lose weight, or to help their hearts, or to firm up their bodies, and kept at it because they discovered that they loved physical exertion. Their stories are legion and the elaborate plans they make to exercise can sound daunting to anyone who is not hooked. But I understand. I plan my days with exercise in them, just as I plan time to eat and sleep, to work, and to spend time with my friends and family.

Exercise makes me feel exhilarated and strong, it makes me feel focused. I understand what Jack LaLanne was getting at when he told me, in words that sound a bit harsh, that he had no patience with people who said they had no time for exercise. "If you can't afford a half-hour two or three times a week to take care of your body, you've got to be sick."

It's Wednesday night at Gold's Gym and Joe Alfano, a young stock trader, and I are chatting between weight-lifting sets as we wait for the 7:30 Spinning class to begin. Joe tells me that while we all hate it when a class starts so late—by the time we get home it's nearly 9:00 p.m.—it's better than the Tuesday and Thursday Spinning classes at 6:30. On those days, he has to leave his office in Manhattan at 4:00 p.m. to catch a subway to Pennsylvania Station. The train ride to New Jersey is nearly an hour, and if the train is late, he cannot make the class. From the train, Joe dashes to his car and drives another fifteen or twenty minutes, depending on traffic on Route 1, to the gym. But to leave the office by 4:00, he has to carefully plan his day, arriving before 8:00 in the morning. And to do that, he has to leave his house in New Jersey before 6:00 a.m. And all for a Spinning class. And all because, he says, he craves the feeling he gets from a vigorous workout. He likes to think he may be healthier, but, he says, he is not doing it primarily for his health. He is doing it for pleasure.

I understand—I do similar things myself and to be sure that I can fit time into my schedule for the exercise I crave, I actually go to three gyms, one in Manhattan and two in New Jersey.

Those who never really enjoyed exercise seldom keep it up. Very few are like Steve Vogel, who hates exercise but keeps coming to his cardiac rehabilitation group's early morning sessions, where he walks and jogs. Most who never felt the joy that exercise can bring make at best halfhearted and sporadic attempts at physical activity. Then they stop altogether, or stay away from it for months at a time, feeling guilty all the while.

A few days after I talk to Joe, I run into Marc Drimmer, a plastic surgeon, climbing onto the elliptical trainer at Gold's Gym. I have not seen him there for months. He tells me he has been busy. His girlfriend was sick; he had to go to a plastic surgeons' convention in Las Vegas. He has an elliptical trainer at home, so I ask him if he has been working out on it. Well, no, he replies. He hasn't had time. "Marc," I say, "do you really like to exercise?" He tells me that, actually, he doesn't. He just thinks that he *should* be exercising.

One day, I get an e-mail from Richard Friedman, the avid swimmer and psychopharmacologist at the Cornell medical school. He knows I'm writing this book and he has a question: "Are you planning to tell the truth about exercise?" he asks me.

I write back. What, I ask, is the truth?

"Ah, the truth about exercise?" he replies. "Well, I suspect that exercise is more often a marker of health than its cause— healthy people like to exercise more than unhealthy people to start with. And the real value of it is not in terms of abstract health benefits like longevity—an extra few hours or maybe months—but because it feels good when you do it or when it's over. To hell with Hygeia; the truth lies in pleasure."

NOTES

one: LESS IS MORE, OR IS IT?

4 **I pick up *Self* magazine** "The #1 Slim-Down Secret," *Self*, August 2001, pp. 120–23.

9 **The College says aerobic endurance training** M. L. Pollack et al., "Position Stand: The Recommended Quantity and Quality of Exercise for Maintaining Cardiorespiratory and Muscular Fitness and Flexibility in Healthy Adults, *Medicine and Science in Sports & Exercise*, vol. 30, no. 6, June 1998, p. 1.

10 **"This was the biggest disappointment of my career"** Gina Kolata, "Studies Find Beta Carotene, Used by Millions, Doesn't Forestall Cancer or Heart Disease," *New York Times*, Jan. 19, 1996, p. A1.

10 **"We deceived ourselves and we deceived our patients"** Gina Kolata and Kurt Eichenwald, "Hope For Sale (A Special Report): Business Thrives on Unproven Care, Leaving Science Behind," *New York Times*, Oct. 3, 1999, p. A1.

18 **"The theory underlying my invention"** U.S. Patent 5752521, Dardik, May 19, 1998, Dardik Therapeutic Exercise Program, p. 5.

18 **"The hunting of animals in the wild"** Ibid., p. 7.

18 **The application goes on to provide "examples of treatment."** Ibid., pp. 10–11.

19 **"an internal wave produced by a biological clock"** U.S. Patent 5810737, Dardik, September 22, 1998, Chronotherapy Exercise Technique, p. 3.

20 **The story emerged in documents** State of New York Department of Health State Board for Professional Conduct, "In the Matter of Irving I. Dardik, M.D., Amended Statement of Charges," November 9, 1994, and "Determination Committee as to Penalty," March 22, 1995; and "In the Matter of Irving I. Dardik, M.D., Administrative Review Decision and Order Number ARB NO. 95–96," October 23, 2000.

two: HISTORY REPEATS ITSELF

26 **"If you read Ken Cooper's** *Aerobics"* Sheehan quoted in James B. Fixx, *The Complete Book of Running* (New York: Random House, 1977), p. 253.

27 **"They gave up mentally before they gave up physically"** Kenneth H. Cooper, *Aerobics* (New York: Bantam Books, 1968), p. 2.

30 **Starting with Herodicus . . . who wrote of "therapeutic gymnastics"** Jack W. Berryman and Roberta J. Park, eds., *Sport and Exercise Science: Essays in the History of Sports Medicine* (Urbana, Illinois: University of Illinois Press, 1992), pp. xi–xii.

30 **something he called "gymnastic medicine"** Jack W. Berryman, "Exercise and the Medical Tradition from Hippocrates Through Antebellum America: A Review Essay," in Berryman and Park, eds., *Sport and Exercise Science*, p. 12.

31 **In** *Regimen in Health,* **Hippocrates** Ibid., p. 13.

31 **Writing in the second century** A.D., **Galen** Ibid., p. 14.

31 **"To me it does not seem that all movement"** From Galen's *On Hygiene*, quoted in Ibid., p. 15.

32 **In the sixteenth century, his writings** Ibid., p. 16.

32 **"To preserve health, we must do our exercises"** Mendez, quoted in Ibid., p. 19.

32 **One such text,** *An Essay of Health and a Long Life* Ibid., p. 30.

33 **"There was no need to run faster"** Peter Radford, "Endurance Runners in Britain before the Twentieth Century," in Dan Tunstall Pedoe, ed., *Marathon Medicine* (London: Royal Society of Medicine Press Ltd., 2000), p. 21.

33 **Some of the men's ages seem exaggerated** Ibid., p. 17.

34 **"because of his 'gross habits of body' "** Ibid., p. 19.

34 **One thin man wore a 58-pound pad** Ibid., p. 19.

34 **"In 1823, a girl of about 11 years"** Ibid., p. 24.

34 **Emma Freedman . . . "the Pedestrian Girl"** Ibid., p. 25.

34 **"attempted to run 96 miles in 24 hours"** Ibid., p. 25.

35 **won in 1809 by Captain Alardice Barclay** Ibid., p. 24.

35 **contests ranging from a 440-yard dash** Ibid., p. 21.

35 **it was thought that they "went rancid in the stomach"** Ibid., p. 27.

35 **The coaches put camphorated oil in their mouths** Ibid., p. 20.

35 **Thom advised starting the day at five a.m.** Roberta J. Park, "Athletes and Their Training in Britain and America, 1800–1914," in Berryman and Park, eds., *Sport and Exercise Science*, pp. 63–64.

36 **Athletic training manuals** Ibid., p. 78.

36 **"Weston the Pedestrian"—won $10,000** Harvey Green, *Fit for America: Health Fitness Sport in American Society* (Baltimore and London: Johns Hopkins University Press, 1986), p. 205.

36 "Much as unqualified 'experts' still purvey their 'systems' " Introduction, Berryman and Park, eds., *Sport and Exercise Science*, p. xvi.

37 "Late Victorian physicians" James C. Whorton, " 'Athlete's Heart': The Medical Debate over Athleticism, 1870–1920," in Berryman and Park, eds., *Sport and Exercise Science*, p. 112.

37 Many used special exercise equipment Green, *Fit for America*, pp. 190–96.

37 women were taking up . . . "purposive exercise" Jan Todd, *Physical Culture and the Body Beautiful: Purposive Exercise in the Lives of American Women, 1800–1875* (Macon, Georgia: Mercer University Press, 1998), p. 3.

37 Some women carried purposive exercise Jan Todd, "Past, Present and Future Perspectives on Strength Training for Female Athletes," Keynote Address, New England Chapter of the American College of Sports Medicine, Concord, Massachusetts, March 2, 2000.

37 In France, a strongwoman named Olga Ibid.

38 In the United States Ibid.

38 "there can be no beauty without fine muscles" Jan Todd, "Bernarr Macfadden: Reformer of Feminine Form," in Berryman and Park, eds., *Sport and Exercise Science*, p. 220.

38 "Weakness is a crime." Ibid., p. 228.

38 "the best and most perfectly formed woman" Ibid., pp. 224–25.

39 The winner, Marie Spitzer Ibid., p. 225.

39 "The old sport died" Radford, "Endurance Runners in Britain," p. 27.

39 He saw "action and sport as a revitalizing agent" Green, *Fit for America*, p. 236.

39 But by the start of the twentieth Peter Radford, "Endurance Runners in Britain Before the Twentieth Century," in Dan Tunstall Pedoe, ed. *Marathon Medicine* (London: Royal Society of Medicine Press Ltd., 2000), pp. 25–26; and Roberta J. Park, "Athletes and Their Training, 1800–1914," in Berryman and Park, eds., *Sport and Exercise Science*, pp. 65–71.

40 "Teddy's Adventures in Africa" Green, *Fit for America*, p. 236.

40 A strongman and trainer Kim Beckwith and Jan Todd, "Requiem for a Strongman: Reassessing the Career of Professor Louis Atilla," *Iron Game History*, July 2002, 7:42–48.

40 "To attract the right kind of clientele" Ibid., p. 47.

40 At first, Attila's clients were men Ibid., p. 48.

40 Attila had disparaged American women Ibid., p. 81.

41 "Actress Edna Wallace Hopper reported" Ibid., p. 82.

41 His most famous female student Ibid., p. 52.

41 Fitness "was a fad" Interview with Jan Todd, July 15, 2002.

41 A paper by Hans Kraus and Ruth Hirschland H. Kraus and R. P. Hirschland, "Muscular Fitness and Health, *Journal for Health, Physical Fitness, and Recreation*, 1953, 24:17–19.

42 **Eisenhower said he was shocked by its findings** "Is American Youth Physically Fit?" *U.S. News and World Report*, Aug. 2, 1957, p. 66.

42 **There were dissenters** Ibid., p. 72.

43 **One of . . . Kennedy's first items of business** *The Surgeon General's Report on Physical Activity and Health*, 1966, chap. 2, p. 18.

44 **" 'Maybe I should do push-ups' "** Interview with Jan Todd, July 16, 2002.

44 **"In the early 1960s, still firm"** Robert Lipsyte, "What Price Fitness," *New York Times Magazine*, Feb. 16, 1986, p. 32.

45 **"Doc, I don't need much endurance"** Cooper, *Aerobics*, p. 11.

45 **"One of the great disappointments"** Ibid., p. 82.

45 **He tells of a Seattle woman** Ibid.

45 **The report stated that just 15 percent** Report of the Surgeon General: *Physical Activity and Health* (www.cdc.gov/nccdphp/sgr/chap5.htm).

46 **a prescription very different from** See Web site of the American Heart Association for recommendations for cardiac rehabilitation (www.aha.org).

46 **"At the age of 45, I . . . got off the train"** George Sheehan, quoted in Andrew Sheehan, *Chasing the Hawk: Looking for My Father, Finding Myself* (New York: Delacorte Press, 2001), p. 79.

46 **His son Andrew wrote** Ibid. pp. 79–80.

47 **"Do your own thing"** Ibid., p. 117.

47 **"what I found even more interesting"** Fixx, *The Complete Book of Running*, p. xviii.

47 **"I am sick of joggers"** Deford, quoted in Sheehan, *Chasing the Hawk*, p. 181.

48 **"I have always made a point"** Jane Fonda, *Jane Fonda's New Workout & Weight-Loss Program* (New York: Simon and Schuster, 1986), p. 89.

48 **Footwear sales rose from $1.8 billion in 1981** "The Sporting Goods Market," a report published annually by the National Sporting Goods Association, Mount Prospect, Illinois.

48 **Exercise classes at health clubs proliferated** "Spanning 20 Years: IDEA and the Fitness Industry," *IDEA Health and Fitness Source*, July–August 2002, pp. 20–21, 28–29, 44–45, 52–53.

48 **Personal trainers became a presence** *IDEA Personal Trainer*, July–August 2002, p. 4; *IDEA Health and Fitness Source*, July–August 2002, p. 53.

three: HOW MUCH IS ENOUGH?

52 **"To most early twentieth-century physicians"** James C. Whorton, " 'Athlete's Heart': The Medical Debate over Athleticism, 1870–1920," in Jack W. Berryman and Roberta J. Park, eds., *Sport and Exercise Science: Essays in the History of Sports Medicine* (Urbana, Illinois: University of Illinois Press, 1992), p. 116.

52 **"Every year, the death rate"** Quoted in Ibid.

52 Whorton recounts some of the alarming stories Ibid., p. 117.

53 "Many have died of heart disease" Quoted in Ibid., p. 120.

53 "Mr. C.," reported a New York physician Ibid.

53 "I feared sudden death" Ibid., p. 121.

53 In 1897, when the Boston Athletic Association Ibid., p. 126.

54 "Pheidippides was more likely" Paul Thompson, "Development of the Marathon from Pheidippides to the Present, with Statistics of Significant Races," *Annals of the New York Academy of Sciences* (301:820–57), 1977.

54 A terrifying story of athlete's heart Whorton, "Athlete's Heart," pp. 120–21.

54 Bicyclists were racing 500 miles in twenty-four hours Ibid., p. 125.

54 Medical experts fretted Ibid., p. 124.

55 Of course, there were skeptics Ibid.

55 Harold Williams and Horace Arnold Ibid., p. 126.

56 "Frequently, the men in the shops" Clarence DeMar, *Marathon: The Clarence DeMar Story* (Tallahassee: Cedarwinds Publishing Company, 1992), p. 6; first published by Stephen Daye Press, 1937.

56 "He [the doctor] told me" Ibid., p. 8.

56 In 1911, he entered the Boston Marathon Ibid., p. 11.

56 In 1912, DeMar stopped running marathons Ibid., p. 36.

58 Cooper advised Americans not to worry Kenneth H. Cooper, *Aerobics* (New York: Bantam Books, 1968), p. 67.

58 His evidence was not exactly scientific Bassler, T. J., letter, Lancet, 2 (1972) 711–12.

59 While many medical experts disputed T. D. Noakers and L. H. Opie, "Heart Diseases in Marathon Runners," *Physician and Sportsmedicine*, vol. 7, no. 11 (November 1979), pp. 141–42.

59 Hal Higdon, a runner Hal Higdon, *Marathon: The Ultimate Training Guide* (Emmaus, Pennsylvania: Rodale Press, 1999), p. 3.

59 In the end, Higdon writes Ibid., pp. 3–4.

60 Jim Fixx, one of the leaders of the running movement Jane Gross, "James F. Fixx Dies Jogging," *New York Times*, July 22, 1984, p. A24.

60 All of the major arteries leading to Fixx's heart Lawrence K. Altman, "The Doctor's World: James Fixx: The Enigma of Heart Disease, *New York Times*, July 24, 1984, p. C1.

60 "The dramatic death of James F. Fixx, guru of exercise fanatics," James A. Michener, "Living with an Ailing Heart," *New York Times Magazine*, Aug. 19, 1984, p. 26.

60 "Longevity is the most compelling" Henry A. Solomon, *The Exercise Myth: A New Approach to Health and Fitness* (New York: Bantam Books, 1984), p. 44.

61 "No one has shown any" Ibid., p. 19.

61 "People with even severe coronary" Ibid., p. 21–22.

61 **Robert Lipsyte reported in 1986** Robert Lipsyte, "What Price Fitness," *New York Times Magazine*, Feb. 16, 1986, p. 32.

62 **Blair reported his results in 1989** S. N. Blair et al., "Physical Fitness and All-Cause Mortality," *Journal of the American Medical Association*, 1989, 262:17:2395–2401.

63 **a study by JoAnn E. Manson** J. E. Manson et al., "A Prospective Study of Walking as Compared with Vigorous Exercise in the Prevention of Coronary Heart Disease in Women," *New England Journal of Medicine*, 1999, 341:650–58.

64 **"Even men who only walked"** R. S. Paffenbarger, "Physical Activity and Coronary Heart Disease in Men: Does the Duration of an Exercise Episode Predict Risk?" *Circulation*, 2000, 102:981–86.

64 **One of the first of these studies** M. Karvonen, K. Kentala, and O. Mustala, "The Effects of Training Heart Rate: A Longitudinal Study," *Annales medicinae experimentalis et biologiae Fenniae*, 1957, 35:307–15.

65 **One, a 1967 study by Brian J. Sharkey** B. J. Sharkey and J. P. Hollerman, "Intensity and Duration of Training and the Development of Cardiorespiratory Endurance," *Medicine and Science in Sports and Exercise*, 1967, 2:197–202.

65 **Another, conducted in 1970 by Irvin Faria** I. E. Faria, "Cardiovascular Response to Exercise as Influenced by Training at Various Intensities," *Research Quarterly for Exercise and Sport*, 1970, 41:41–50.

66 **"Lack of statistically significant findings"** S. N. Blair and J. C. Connelly, "How Much Physical Activity Should We Do? The Case for Moderate Amounts and Intensities of Physical Activity," *Research Quarterly for Exercise and Sport*, 1996, 67:2:198.

66 **How little can you do** Roy J. Shephard and Gary J. Balady, "Exercise as Cardiovascular Therapy," *Circulation*, 1999, 99:963–72; and Michael L. Pollock et al., "Position Stand. The Recommended Quantity and Quality of Exercise for Developing and Maintaining Cardiorespiratory and Muscular Fitness, and Flexibility in Healthy Adults," *Medicine and Science in Sports and Exercise*, 1998, 30:6.

68 **60 percent of the population gets no regular exercise** U.S. Department of Health and Human Services, *Physical Activity and Health: A Report of the Surgeon General* (Atlanta: U.S. Department of Health and Human Services, Centers for Disease Control and Prevention, National Center for Chronic Disease Prevention and Health Promotion, 1996); and CDC's report *Healthy People 2010* (www.health.gov/healthypeople/document/html/objectives/22-01.htm).

four: MAXIMUM HEART RATES
       AND FAT-BURNING ZONES

80 **"Lance is never far from his heart-rate monitor"** Lance Armstrong and Chris Carmichael, *The Lance Armstrong Performance Program* (Emmaus, Pennsylvania: Rodale Press, 2000), p. 59.

83 **Their paper, published in 1970** S. M. Fox and W. L. Haskell, "Detection of Coronary Heart Disease as a Challenge to the Work Physiologist," in *Research Conference on Applied Work Physiology* (New York: New York University Medical Center, 1970).

84 **The two presented the graph at another meeting** S. M. Fox and W. L. Haskell, "The Exercise Stress Test: Needs for Standardization," in M. Eliskim and H. N. Neufeld, eds., *Cardiology: Current Topics and Progress* (New York: Academic Press, 1970), pp. 149–56.

84 **At yet another meeting that year** S. M. Fox and W. L. Haskell, "Detection of Coronary Heart Disease as a Challenge to the Work Physiologist," in *Research Conference on Applied Work Physiology* (1970).

84 **Finally, in 1971, Fox and Haskell** S. M. Fox, J. P. Naughton, and W. L. Haskell, "Physical Activity and the Prevention of Coronary Heart Disease," *Annals of Clinical Research*, 1971, 3:404–32.

87 **Seals reported that a person's maximum heart rate** H. Tanaka, K. D. Monahan, and D. R. Seals, "Age-Predicted Heart Rate Revisited," *Journal of the American College of Cardiology*, 2001, 37:1:153–58.

90 **"This is not an easy test," writes Lance Armstrong's trainer** Armstrong and Carmichael, *The Lance Armstrong Performance Program*, pp. 62–63.

90 **John L. Parker, Jr., a runner** John L. Parker, Jr., *Heart Rate Monitor Training for the Compleat Idiot* (Medway, Ohio: Cedarwinds Publishing Company, 1993), pp. 19–21.

91 **The American College of Sports Medicine advises** D. A. Mahler et al., eds., *ACSM's Guidelines for Exercise Testing and Prescription*, fifth edition, (Philadelphia: A. Waverly Company, 1995), p. 25.

91 **The American College of Cardiology** R. J. Gibbons et al., "ACC/AHA Guidelines for Exercise Testing," *American Journal of Cardiology*, 1997, 30:260–315.

91 **The biggest risk is that atherosclerotic plaque** S. Giri, P. D. Thompson, F. J. Kiernan, et al., "Clinical and Angiographic Characteristics of Exercise-related Acute Myocardial Infarction," *Journal of the American Medical Association*, 1999, 282:1731–36.

91 **In his 1993 paper . . . Mittleman** M. A. Mittleman et al., "Triggering of Acute Myocardial Infarction by Heavy Physical Exertion—Protection Against Triggering by Regular Exertion," *New England Journal of Medicine*, 1993, 329:23:1677–83.

91 **Others investigated the risk of sudden death** C. M. Albert et al., "Trigger-

ing of Sudden Death from Cardiac Causes by Vigorous Exertion," *New England Journal of Medicine*, 2000, 343:9:1355–61.

96 **That certainly is true for diets** R. L. Leibel, J. Hirsch, B. E. Appel, and G. C. Checani, "Energy Intake Required to Maintain Body Weight Is Not Affected by Wide Variation in Diet Composition," *American Journal of Clinical Nutrition*, 1992, 55:350–55.

98 **"The total calories from fat"** Jack H. Wilmore and David L. Costill, *Physiology of Sport and Exercise*, second edition (Champaign, Illinois: Human Kinetics, 1999), p. 682.

five: TRAINING LORE

105 **The Boston Athletic Association has** (www.bostonmarathon.org/marathon training.htm).

105 **Hal Higdon, who trains** (www.halhigdon.com/marathon).

107 **"I eat food," he said, "I don't taste it."** Blaine Harden, "For a Speed Hiker, Three Trails End in Maine and a Record," *New York Times*, Oct. 27, 2001.

107 **For bicycling, I find some very odd training advice** Joel Friel, *The Cyclist's Training Bible: A Complete Training Guide for the Competitive Cyclist* (Boulder, Colorado: VeloPress, 1996), p. 15.

107 **Clarence DeMar, the champion marathon runner** Clarence DeMar, *Marathon: The Clarence DeMar Story* (Tallahassee, Florida: Cedarwinds Publishing Co., 1992), pp. 5–6; first published by Stephen Daye Press, 1937.

108 **On the day of the Boston Marathon** Ibid., p. 15.

108 **One of the greatest runners ever . . . Emil Zapotek** "Horrible Extremities of Pain" (www.angelfire.com/rock/running/essays/evolution5.html).

108 **Another legendary runner** Trishul Cherns, "Ted Corbitt: An Ultrarunning Pioneer," *Ultrarunning Magazine Online* (www.ultrarunning.com/archives/corbitt.htm).

109 **"It was a snowy February day"** Ted Corbitt, "A Willingness to Suffer," in Gail Waesche Kislevitz, *First Marathons: Personal Encounters with the 26.2 Mile Monster* (Halcottsville, N.Y.: Breakaway Books, 1998), p. 82.

110 **In 1977, Ron Richardson** David Samuel, "The Runner," *New Yorker*, Sept. 3, 2001, p. 81.

111 **What is possibly the ultimate in training stories** Bernd Heinrich, *Why We Run: A Natural History* (New York: HarperCollins, Ecco pbk., 2002).

111 **Heinrich was no novice** Ibid., p. 17.

111 **"I had to remodel myself"** Ibid., p. 198.

111 **He asked himself how he would get enough fuel** Ibid., p. 223.

111 **"That was frightening."** Ibid., p. 229.

112 **He also worried about endurance** Ibid., p. 231.

112 **Now there was the problem of what to eat** Ibid., pp. 213–18.

112 **Looking still to animals** Ibid., p. 235.

113 **He won. Still, in retrospect** Ibid., p. 264.

114 **Rendell and Gerschler decided to try something different** Amby Burfoot, "Runner's World: Training and Racing" (www.angelfire.com/rock/running/essays/evolution4.html).

114 **To demonstrate the value of their method** Ibid., p. 2.

115 **As Bannister drew close to the finish line** Roger Bannister, "The Four Minute Mile!" (http://faculty.rmwc.edu/tmichalik/4min.htm).

115 **His coach was Franz Stampfl** Ibid., p. 6.

117 **Cortland's yearbook** *The Didascaleion* (Cortland, N.Y.: SUNY Cortland, 1965), p. 164.

120 **Duke University biologist Steven Vogel** Steven Vogel, *Prime Mover: A Natural History of Muscle* (New York: W.W. Norton, 2001), p. 16.

122 **"It was the first time anyone had taken muscles"** Lawrence C. Rome et al., "Why Animals Have Different Vire Types," *Nature*, 1998, 335:6193:824–27.

125 **His device changed all that** S. Salmons, "An implantable Muscle Stimulator," *Journal of Physiology*, 1967, 188:13–14.

125 **When he did the critical experiment** S. Salmons and G. Vrbová, "The Influence of Activity on Some Contractile Characteristics of Mammalian Fast and Slow Muscles," Ibid., 1969, 201:535–49.

125 **"That paper, published in *Nature* in 1976"** S. Salmons and F. A. Sréter, "Significance of Impulse Activity in the Transformation of Skeletal Muscle Type," *Nature*, 1976, 263:30–34.

126 **With exercise the main changes** S. Salmons, "Section 7: Muscle," in P. L. Williams et al., eds., *Gray's Anatomy* (New York, Edinburgh, London, Tokyo, Madrid, Melbourne: Churchill Livingstone, 1995), pp. 737–900.

130 **One measurement of a training response** Claude Bouchard et al., "Familial Aggregation of VO2mas Response to Exercise Training: Results from the HERITAGE Family Study," *Journal of Applied Physiology*, 1999, 87:1003–8.

130 **One analysis of fifty-nine studies** Z. V. Tran and A. Weltman, "Differential Effects of Exercise on Serum Lipid and Lipoprotein Levels Seen with Changes in Body Weight: A Meta-analysis," *Journal of the American Medical Association*, 1985, 254:919–24.

six: THE ATHLETE'S WORLD

136 **He recalled those awful days of the race** Johnny G and Andrea Cagan, *Romancing the Bicycle: The Five Spokes of Balance* (Los Angeles: Johnny G Publishing Co., 2000), p. 14.

136 **"I vaguely remember"** Ibid.

136 "A fellow rider told me" Ibid., p. 16.

136 "So why am I doing this?" Ibid.

137 "Satan says I have to pedal" Ibid., p. 23.

137 "When an athlete learns" Ibid., p. 62.

138 "three very slippery drums" Ibid., p. 8.

138 "The stationary bike would no longer exist" Ibid., p. 9.

139 "Even if you choose" Ibid., p. 75.

139 "My goal for the Spinning program" Ibid., p. 10.

142 he thought of himself as "bridging the gap" Robert Massie and Suzanne Massie, *Journey: The Classic Story of a Son's Illness and a Family's Courage* (New York: Ballantine Books, 1984), p. 353.

143 "I would think of Jamie as he swam" Ibid., p. 352.

144 "It got to the point . . . 'The Untouchables' " *The Didascaleion* (Cortland, N.Y.: SUNY Cortland, 1965), p. 164.

seven: MOUNT EVEREST

163 In one study, published in 1980 D. L. Costill and J. M. Miller, "Nutrition for Endurance Sport: Carbohydrate and Fluid Balance," *International Journal of Sports Medicine*, 1980, 1:2–14.

163 In another study, published in 1988 D. L. Costill, "Nutrition for Sports Performance," in E. R. Burke and M. N. Newsome, eds., *Medical and Scientific Aspects of Cycling: Proceedings of 1986 World Congress*, 1988, pp. 25–37.

165 "It was a stupid rule" D. L. Costill, W. F. Kammer, and A. Fisher, "Fluid Ingestion During Distance Running," *Archives of Environmental Health*, 1970, 21:520–25.

166 Some extreme examples of the problem of drinking *Annals of the New York Academy of Sciences*, 1977, 301:183–88.

eight: IS THERE A RUNNER'S HIGH?

175 I glance at a popular bodybuilding magazine Ben Kaller, "Conquer Your Food Cravings," *Men's Fitness*, Feb. 2002, p. 82.

176 "And I feel wonderful" Sherwin B. Nuland, "Aging Bulls Buff Up, and Build Bones, Too," *New York Times*, Feb. 17, 1999, p. G14.

176 "helping your brain experience pleasure" From the Web site of the Chemical Heritage Foundation (www.chemheritage.org).

177 Cornell University's nutrition division Nutriquest may be accessed through the university's Web site (www.nutrition.cornell.edu).

178 "At first, the tobacco and smoke" William P. Morgan, "Negative Addiction in Runners," *The Physician and Sportsmedicine*, 1979, 7:2:57–69.

178 He provides some . . . case studies Ibid., pp. 67–69.

186 **The great English doctor, Thomas Sydenham** Lubert Stryer, *Biochemistry* (San Francisco: W.H. Freeman, 1975), p. 851.

187 **The first clue came in 1975** Ibid., p. 852.

193 **The same thing happens with running** B. T. Lett et al., "Pairings of a Distinctive Chamber with the Aftereffect of Wheel Running Produce Conditioned Place Preference," *Appetite*, 2000, 34:87–94.

193 **Neuroscientist Stefan Brene and his colleagues** M. Werme et al., "Running Increases Ethanol Preference," *Behavioral Brain Research*, 2000, 1–8.

194 **But the same phenomenon** B. T. Lett et al., "Wheel Running Simultaneously Produces Conditioned Taste Aversion and Conditioned Place Preference in Rats," *Learning and Motivation*, 2001, 32:129–36.

195 **Brene . . . focused on Lewis rats** M. Werme et al., "Addiction-Prone Lewis but Not Fischer Rats Develop Compulsive Running That Coincides with Downregulation of Nerve Growth Factor Inducible-B and Neuron-Derived Orphan Receptor 1," *Journal of Neuroscience*, 1999, 19:6169–74.

196 **He looked at the production of enkephalin** M. Werme et al., "Running and Cocaine Both Upregulate Dynorphin mRNA in Medial Cudate Putamen," *European Journal of Neuroscience*, 2000, 12:2967–74.

199 **After four months, the investigators found** J. A. Blumenthal et al., "Effects of Exercise Training on Older Patients with Major Depression," *Archives of Internal Medicine*, 1999, 195:2349–56.

nine: SCULPTING THE BODY BEAUTIFUL

209 **weight lifting "had a negative image"** John D. Fair, *Muscletown USA: Bob Hoffman and the Manly Culture of York Barbell* (University Park, Pennsylvania: Pennsylvania State University Press, 1999), p. 2.

210 **Hoffman published books . . . such as *Broad Shoulders*** Ibid., p. 108.

210 **the archetypical Horatio Alger story** Ibid., p. 2.

210 **One of Hoffman's lifters, Dick Bachtell,** Ibid., p. 44.

211 **"It was pitched to the middle-class belief"** Ibid., p. 50.

211 **"Grimek became an inspiration"** Ibid., p. 63.

211 **Vic Tanny, who went on to found** Ibid., p. 126.

212 **"The greatest muscle picture ever shown"** Ibid., p. 109.

212 **"As for myself, I almost live on Hi-Proteen."** Ibid., p. 149.

212 **He promised that his diets and supplements** Ibid., p. 193.

213 **"Unsure of the results it would produce"** Ibid., p. 207.

213 **Senator Edward Long of Missouri** Ibid., p. 207.

214 **He had hired a local blacksmith** Marla Matzer Rose, Muscle Beach (New York: St. Martin's Press, 2001), p. 59.

214 **One of Muscle Beach's most famous** Ibid., p. 46.

214 **Her boyfriend, later husband, Les Stockton** Ibid., p. 49.

215 **She was featured in photo essays** Jan Todd, "Abbye 'Pudgy' Stockton," in

Tom Pendergast and Sara Pendergast, eds. *St. James Encyclopedia of Popular Culture*, 5 vols. (Framington Hills, Mich.: St. James Press, 1999), p. 541.

215 **The phenomenon that was Muscle Beach** Ibid., pp. 128–30.

215 **"The Birthplace of the Fitness Boom"** Ibid., p. 1.

215 **Hoffman had largely shut Weider** Fair, *Muscletown USA*, p. 5.

215 **Weider was a teenage wonder** See Web site of the International Federation of Bodybuilders (www.ifbb.com/joe).

215 **In 1939, while still a scrawny** Rose, *Muscle Beach*, p. 214.

216 **"I asked myself, How many guys"** Ibid., p. 196.

216 **He moved to Union City . . . in 1947** Ibid., pp. 197–98.

216 **Dr. Frederick Tilney from Hollywood** Fair, *Muscletown USA*, p. 129.

216 **Weider created a "Weider Research Clinic"** Ibid.

216 **It was Orlick who conceived** Ibid., p. 128.

217 **"A *boobybuilder* is usually"** Ibid., p. 169.

217 **Weider fought back, attacking Hoffman** Ibid., pp. 177–78.

219 **"What had enabled Hoffman"** Ibid., p. 350.

220 **Steroids were developed in the 1930s** Ibid., p. 195.

220 **A doctor, John Ziegler** Ibid.

220 **In 1971, one of Hoffman's lifters, Ken Patera** Terry Todd, "Anabolic Steroids and Sport," in Jack W. Berryman and Roberta K. Park, eds., *Sport and Exercise Science: Essays in the History of Sports Medicine* (Urbana, Illinois: University of Illinois Press, 1992), p. 326.

220 **"Some go so far as to say"** Ibid., p. 278.

221 **"Those on the 'inside' knew"** Ibid., p. 280.

221 **one California doctor, Walter F. Jekot** Todd, "Anabolic Steroids and Sport," p. 350.

222 **She became a celebrity** Fair, *Muscletown USA*, p. 359.

223 **One woman . . . Tammy Thompson** Ibid., pp. 320–21.

223 **In 1981, NBC sports announcer Mike Adamle** Ibid., p. 344.

224 **"Muscular fitness is of some value"** Kenneth H. Cooper, *Aerobics* (New York: Bantam Books, 1968), p. 13.

224 **He had been an artist's model** Jan Todd, "Bodybuilding," in Tom Pendergast and Sara Pendergast, eds., *St. James Encyclopedia of Popular Culture*, 5 vols. (Framington Hills, Mich.: St. James Press, 1999), pp. 305–8.

225 **Hoffman took Atlas on** Fair, *Muscle Beach*, p. 56.

226 **The allures of strength training were on display** "The Evolution of the Personal Trainer," *ACE Fitness Matters*, Jan.–Feb. 2002, pp. 6–7.

230 **"Randomized clinical trials of exercise"** NIH Consensus Development Panel on Osteoporosis Prevention, Diagnosis, and Therapy, "Osteoporosis Prevention, Diagnosis, and Therapy," *Journal of the American Medical Association*, 2001, 285:6:786.

233 **Jane Fonda, for example, told women** Jane Fonda, *Jane Fonda's New*

Workout & Weight Loss Program (New York: Simon and Schuster, 1986), pp. 114 and 190.

235 **The accumulated knowledge to date** William J. Kraemer et al., ACSM Position Stand, Feb. 1, 2002: "Progression Models in Resistance Training for Healthy Adults" (see "Position Stands" at www.acsm-msse.org).

ten: THE FITNESS BUSINESS

242 **The ACE Web site did not reveal** (www.acefitness.org).

245 **At least one organization, the American College of Sports Medicine** www.acsm.org.

247 **At its meeting in Miami** ECA Miami 2002 Sports Training & Fitness Conference brochure.

248 **"Responses were below"** Dixie Stanforth, Philip R. Stanforth, and Margaret F. Hoemeke, "Physiologic and Metabolic Responses to a Body Pump Workout," *Journal of Strength and Conditioning Research*, 2000, 14:2:144–50.

250 **Its inventor, Ken Hutchins, says** See the Web site of the SuperSlow Exercise Guild (www.superslow.com).

250 **The ACE magazine for personal trainers** Jim Gerard, "SuperSlow: One Man's Defiant Challenge," *ACE Fitnessmatters*, March–April 2002, pp. 7–9.

251 **One group at George Washington University** Laura K. Keeler et al., "Early-Phase Adaptations of Traditional-Speed vs. Superslow Resistance Training on Strength and Aerobic Capacity in Sedentary Individuals," *Journal of Strength and Conditioning Research*, 2001, 15:3:309–14.

251 **"I don't like quoting research papers"** Gerard, "SuperSlow: One Man's Defiant Challenge," p. 8.

251 **Of course, there is a certification process** See the Web site of the SuperSlow Exercise Guild (www.superslow.com).

252 **"While Hutchins claims his protocol"** Gerard, "SuperSlow: One Man's Defiant Challenge," pp. 8–9.

253 **"That was the turning point"** Johnny G and Andrea Cagan, *Romancing the Bicycle: The Five Spokes of Balance* (Los Angeles: Johnny G Publishing Co., 2000), p. 9.

253 **more than 17,000 health clubs** See "Industry Statistics" at the Web site of International Health, Racquet & Sportsclub Association (www.ihrsa.org).

253 **The National Sporting Goods Association** See "Research and Statistics/ Consumer Purchases by Category" at the Web site of National Sporting Goods Association (www.nsga.org).

254 **"many shoe manufacturers are purporting"** Trevor Prior, "New Modalities in the Management of Running Injuries," in Dan Tunstall Pedoe, ed., *Marathon Medicine* (London: Royal Society of Medicine Press Ltd., 2000), p. 314.

254 "It is easy to demonstrate" Ibid.

254 Shoe manufacturers use video Ibid., p. 315.

254 "Detailed mechanism of injury" Martyn Shorten, "Running Shoe Design: Protection and Performance," in Pedoe, ed., *Marathon Medicine*, p. 163.

255 "delicious meal replacement food bar" *Men's Fitness*, March 2002, p. 89.

255 "jolt your metabolism" Ibid., p. 90.

255 The ad does not mention See various warnings of the U.S. Food and Drug Administration (www.fda.gov/ohrms/dockets/dailys/00/mar00/032200/c003699.pdf; and www.cfsan.fda.gov/~lrd/form1.html; and www.cfsan.fda.gov/~dms/ds-ephed.html).

255 "slow-release protein complexes" *Men's Fitness*, March 2002, pp. 120–22.

256 advertisement for a "Ripping Gel" Ibid., p. 103.

258 "Call for a list of physicians" Ibid., p. 145.

258 As evidence that growth hormone D. Rudman et al., "Effects of Human Growth Hormone on Men Over 60 Years Old," *New England Journal of Medicine*, 1990, 323:1:1–6.

258 It involved fifty-two elderly men M. A. Papadakis et al., "Growth Hormone Replacement in Healthy Older Men Improves Body Composition But Not Functional Ability," *Annals of Internal Medicine*, 1996, 124:708–16.

ACKNOWLEDGMENTS

I set out to learn about fitness, exercise, and health knowing I would need help from many medical and scientific experts and ordinary people. I discovered that the patience, thoughtfulness, and generosity of those I contacted knew no bounds. Virtually every living person mentioned in this book deserves my thanks for their gracious assistance.

In addition, I would like to extend special thanks to a few individuals who spent an extraordinary amount of time and effort answering my questions and helping me to check facts, and who provided uniquely valuable perspectives and resources. They include historians John Fair and Jan Todd, exercise physiologists Steve Blair, Dave Costill, Bill Haskell, and William Kraemer, cardiologists Mike Lauer and Paul Thompson, psychopharmacologist Richard Friedman, and obesity researcher and geneticist Claude Bouchard. I am grateful to my friends, who readily agreed to let me tell their stories, and especially to Cynthia.

I also thank my agent, John Brockman, who suggested that I write a book about exercise, and my editor, John Glusman, who saw what this book could be and whose insightful suggestions were an invaluable guide in shaping its content and tone. Finally, I thank my husband, Bill, who listened patiently as I endlessly discussed the book, who offered helpful comments, and who read draft after draft.

INDEX

Adamle, Mike, 224
addiction to exercise, 135, 175, 177–79, 186, 192–97
adenosine triphosphate (ATP), 256–57
aerobics, 6, 9–10, 25–26, 28–29, 48
Aerobics (Cooper), 25–26, 45, 224
aging, 86, 123
Ahrens, Pete, 96–97
Akil, Huda, 189–91
Alexeev, Vasily, 220
Alfano, Joe, 68, 266–67
Amateur Athletic Union, 216, 217, 219
American College of Cardiology, 91
American College of Sports Medicine, 9–10, 91, 235, 245, 263
American Council on Exercise (ACE), 241, 242, 245, 246, 247, 250
American Heart Association, 91
American Journal of Cardiology, 87
American Journal of Clinical Nutrition, 96
American Physical Education Review, 55
anaerobic zone, 79–80, 81
Annals of Internal Medicine, 258
Apex diet/exercise program, 254–55

Armstrong, Lance, 35, 80, 149
Arnold, Horace, 55
athletes: discovery of new talent, 143–46; professional's life, 146–48; special world of, 141–43
"athlete's heart" syndrome, 51–57, 72
Atlas, Charles, 224–25
Attila, Louis, 40–41

Bachtell, Dick, 210
Bannister, Roger Gilbert, 115
Barclay, Alardice, 35, 106
Barnhard, Sue, 135, 139, 168, 170
Barron, Gayle, 102
Bassler, Thomas J., 58–59
Baumann, Carolyn, 41
Beauty and Health magazine, 38
Beauty of Running, The (Barron and Chapin), 102
Benson, Herbert, 12
Berger, Jessica, 248–49
Berger, Richard, 227
Berryman, Jack, 29, 30, 31, 36
bicycling, 37, 73–74, 262; aerobics and, 28; dangers of, 157; heart effects, 54–55; heart-rate determination with, 90; with rollers, 138;

bicycling (*cont.*)
  runner's high from, 179–81, 183;
  Taylor's experiences, 145–48; track
  races, 144–45; training for, 107.
  See also Spinning
Bicycling magazine, 107
Blaikie, William, 54
Blair, Steven N., 51, 62–63, 64–65,
  66, 69–70, 262, 264
Blumenthal, James, 198–200
Body Attack exercise program, 248
Bodyblade workout tool, 249–50
bodybuilding/bodysculpting, 203–5,
  207, 208–9, 213–17, 219, 225
Body Pump exercise program, 247–48
Bodysculpting exercise program, 203
Book of Bodily Exercise (Mendez),
  32
Boston Athletic Association, 105
Boston Medical Journal, 52, 55
Bouchard, Claude, 127–31, 230, 231,
  263
Brene, Stefan, 193, 194, 195–96, 197
Brown, Richard, 33
Bruno, Sam and Kathy, 104, 133
Burke, Edmund, 144
Butterfield, Lady, 34

Cantor, Arnold, 171, 181–82, 259
carbohydrate loading, 112–13, 162–
  63
Carmichael, Chris, 35, 80, 90
Carson, Johnny, 222
Chapin, Kim, 102
Chemical Heritage Foundation, 176–
  77
Cheyne, George, 32
Circulation (journal), 64
Claremont, Alan, 167
cocaine, 180, 183, 195, 196–97
Complete Book of Running, The
  (Fixx), 47
Cooper, Kenneth H., 25–29, 45–46,
  48, 51, 57–58, 61, 67, 70, 224

Corbitt, Ted, 108–10, 119, 164
Cornaccio, Corey, 88
Costill, David, 26, 70–71, 98, 109,
  110, 113, 116–17, 118–19, 127,
  143–45, 158–65, 227
creatine supplements, 256–57
cross-training, 105, 106

D'Andrea, Gregg, 7–8, 9
Dardik, Alison Godfrey, 17, 22
Dardik, Irving, 12–14, 16, 18–21,
  22–23
death during exercise, 60, 91–92, 157
Deford, Frank, 47
Degas, Edgar, 38
DeMar, Clarence, 55–57, 107–8
depression and exercise, 197–200
Desbonnet, Edmund, 37
DeVesley, Jane, 222
diabetes, 187, 232, 263
diet/exercise programs, 254–55
Diseases of Modern Life (Richard-
  son), 52–53
dopamine, 186, 194–95, 196
Doughty, Tom, 144, 145
Dow, Lisa Sherman, 244
Drake, Debbie, 43
Drewnowski, Adam, 175–76
Drimmer, Marc, 267

ECA World Fitness, 247
Eccles, Jack, 125
Eisenhower, Dwight D., 42
encyclopedia.com, 176
endorphins, 173; discovery of, 186–
  88; runner's high and, 175–77,
  188–91, 200; source of, 189
endurance training, 117–18
Essay of Health and a Long Life, An
  (Cheyne), 32
euphoria of exercise, 5, 93, 147–48,
  172–73. *See also* runner's high
Evans, Janet, 4
Evans, Linda, 226

Evolutions Fitness, 133–35, 258–59
Exercise, Etc. company, 247
Exercise Myth, The (Solomon), 60–61

Fair, John D., 207–8, 209, 210, 211, 213, 214, 216, 219, 220, 225
fan use during exercise, 165–66
Faria, Irvin, 65–66
fat-burning zones, 73, 80, 93–99
Federal Trade Commission, 212
Fisher, Irving, 53
Fittrek exercise program, 247
Fitts, Bob, 144
Fixx, Jim, 47, 224; death of, 60, 61
fluid intake, 35, 36, 109, 112; dangers of insufficient intake, 166–67; water needs during exercise, 164–65, 166
Fonda, Jane, 48, 233
Food and Drug Administration (FDA), 212, 213, 255, 258
food intake, 35; diet/exercise programs, 254–55; for marathon running, 107–8, 109, 112–13; nutritional supplements, 210, 212–13, 255–57; for Spinning, 156, 158; sugar to reduce muscle fatigue, 162–64; for walking at competitive level, 107; weight control and, 96–97
Ford, Harrison, 226
Fox, Bill, 156–57, 171, 175, 179–81, 186, 196
Fox, Edward L., 110
Fox, Sam, 83, 84
Frazier, Claire, 96
Freedman, David, 14, 15
Freedman, Emma, 34
Friedman, Richard, 172, 179, 197–98, 200–201, 207, 267

Gajda, Bob, 216
Galen, 31–32

Gallagher, J. Christopher, 229, 230
Gambrell, Larry, 204–6, 240
genetics: muscle response to weight lifting and, 228–29; of runner's high, 191–92, 196; training responsiveness and, 126–31
Gerschler, Woldemar, 114–15
Giro d'Italia race, 258–59
Gold, Joe, 214
Goldberger, Ary, 12, 13, 22–23
Goldman, Denise, 208–9
Gold's Gym, 6, 214, 247–48, 254–55
Goldsmith, Rochelle, 12
Gordon, Erynn, 229
Grant, Virginia, 192, 193, 194
Greeks and Romans, 30–32, 53–54
Green, Harvey, 39
Grimek, John, 211–12, 220
Guillemin, Roger, 187

Hagerman, Fritz, 82–83, 113, 114–16
Hamilton, Linda, 226
Harbig, Rudolph, 114–15
Haskell, William, 83–84, 86, 88
HDL, 130
health-club industry, 226–27, 253
health improvement through exercise, 61–68, 262–65, 267
heart disease, 45–46, 51–57, 65, 91
heart effects of exercise: moderate exercise as best for health, 61–68; vigorous exercise as beneficial for heart, 57–61, 64–65; vigorous exercise as damaging to heart, 51–57, 60–61, 71–72, 91–92
heart rate, 8; aging and, 86; anaerobic zone, 79–80, 81; commercialization of heart-rate information, 88–89; determining one's own maximum rate, 89–92; fat-burning zones, 73, 80, 93–99; formulas for calculating maximum rate, 73, 78–88, 89; as measure of effort, 78;

heart rate (*cont.*)
    monitoring of, 77–79, 80, 88–89, 149; physiology of, 82–83; practical uses for heart-rate information, 86; reliability of data on, 84–86; runner's high and, 180; Spinning and, 73, 77–79, 151; treadmill test for, 80
Heart Waves program, 12–23, 259
Heinrich, Bernd, 111–13, 117, 131
Hennenkens, Charles, 10
Herodicus, 30–31
Herodotus, 54
Hess, Anna, 76, 103, 127, 171
Higdon, Hal, 59, 105–6
High Protein Recipe Book (Hoffman), 212
Hippocrates, 31
Hirsch, Jules, 96–97
Hirschland, Ruth, 41–42
history of exercise and fitness, 29–49; anti-exercise mentality, 44–46; exercise/fitness movement, 46–49; Greeks and Romans, 30–32; "improvement," focus on, 36–41; national security concerns, 41–43; training, 35–36; wagering contests, 32–35, 36, 39
Hoberman, John, 185
Hoffman, Bob, 209–13, 216, 217, 219, 220, 225
Hoffman, Eric, 228
homosexuals, 219
hormone replacement therapy, 264
Hortobagyi, Gabriel, 10
How to Keep Your Husband Happy (Drake), 43
Hughes, John, 187
human growth hormone, 257–58
Hutchins, Ken, 250, 251–52

IDEA organization, 48
International Federation of Body Builders, 216

International Health, Racquet & Sportsclub Association, 253
International Journal of Sports Medicine, 163
interval training, 105, 113–17, 129
Isaacson, Dan, 226
Is Your Child Physically Fit? (Pruden), 42

Jekot, Walter F., 221
Johnny G, 135, 136–39, 140, 149–50, 246, 247, 253
Journal of Orthopedic Sports Physical Therapy, 249
Journal of Strength and Conditioning Research, 248, 251
Journal of the American Medical Association, 53, 62, 230
Journey (Massie), 142

Karpovich, Peter V., 42
Karvonen, Martti, 65
Kennedy, John F., 43
Kirkendall, Donald, 81–82, 83, 85, 93, 117–18, 171, 265–66
Klibanski, Anne, 230
Klugman, Jack, 222
Koob, George, 184–86
Kraemer, William, 219–20, 227, 233–34, 235, 236–37, 263
Kraus, Hans, 41–42

LaForge, Sharon, 134–36, 139–41, 153, 157, 164, 168, 170
LaLanne, Jack, 43, 208, 214, 226, 266
Lauer, Michael, 64, 67, 262–63
Leibel, Rudolph, 96–97
less-is-more movement, 8–23
Lett, Bow Tong, 193, 194
life extension through exercise, 263–64
LifeWaves International, 16–18, 21, 22

Lipsyte, Robert, 44, 61
Lohli, Arline, 92, 94–95, 102, 103
Long, Edward, 213
Lugrin, George, 220–21
Lydiard, Arthur, 116

Macfadden, Bernarr, 38, 39, 224
Mad Dogg Athletics, 151, 245, 246
Manson, JoAnn E., 63, 92
Marathon (DeMar), 56–57
marathon running, 70; fluid intake for, 109, 112, 164–65, 166–67; food intake for, 107–8, 109, 112–13; heart effects, 53–54, 55, 56–57, 58–59; personality for, 109; training for, 105–6, 107–13
Massie, Bob, 142–43
Massie, Robert and Suzanne, 142
McDonald's, 133
McLeod, Donald, 33
McQuillen, Eleanor N., 60
Medical and Scientific Aspects of Cycling, 163
Medicine and Science in Sports, 65
Mendez, Christobal, 32
Men's Fitness magazine, 175, 255, 257
metabolism, 230–32
Meylan, George, 55
Michener, James A., 60
Mittleman, Murray, 91
moderate exercise as best for health, 61–68, 262–63
Moens, Roger, 114
Monohan, Gene, 249
Morgan, William P., 177–78
motives for exercising, 68–71, 262–67
Mount Everest ride, 76–77, 131, 133, 246; "bridging the gap" between athletes and non-athletes, 141–43; ride itself, 167–72; Taylor's inspiration for, 151–53; training for, 101–2, 155–58, 167

Muscle & Fitness magazine, 225
Muscle Beach phenomenon, 213–15
muscles: aging and, 123; beauty and, 38, 204; creatine supplements and, 256–57; fat burning and, 94; fatigue in, 162–64; heart rate and, 82; metabolism and, 230–32; science of building muscles, 227–29; soreness in, 232–33; speed/power trade-off, 122–23; stretching before exercise, 232; training to alter muscle physiology, 119–26; types of muscle fibers, 120–23, 161. *See also* weight lifting
Muscletown USA (Fair), 209

nasal strips, 168
National Police Gazette, 41
National Sporting Goods Association, 253
National Strength and Conditioning Association, 263
Nature magazine, 125
Nautilus company, 250
New England Journal of Medicine, 63, 91, 92, 258
Newkirk, Emma, 38–39
New York City Road Runners Club, 106
New York Medical Journal, 53
New York Times, 176
Nicholson, Jack, 226
Nissen, Steve, 80, 104
Nixon, Richard M., 42
Nuland, Sherwin B., 176
Nutriquest service, 177
nutritional supplements, 210, 212–13, 255–57

Olga (strongwoman), 37–38
On Hygiene (Galen), 31–32
opiates, 186
orgasms, 188
Orlick, E. M., 216

O'Shea, Patrick, 227
osteoporosis, 229–30

Paffenbarger, Ralph S., 64
Park, Jim, 212
Park, Roberta J., 36
Parker, John L., Jr., 90
parlor gymnasium, 37
Pasternak, Gavril, 188–89, 190
Patera, Ken, 220
Pedestrianism (Thom), 35–36
Perrault, Bill, 151, 153, 155, 168,
    169, 170, 171, 258
personal trainers, 3, 48–49, 239–40;
    certification of, 240–46, 251–52;
    conventions for, 246–47
Pheidippides, 53–54
Philadelphia Medical Journal, 55
Physical Culture magazine, 38
"Physical Fitness and All-Cause Mor-
    tality" (Blair), 262, 264
Physician and Sportsmedicine, 72
pleasure of exercise, 207–9, 266–
    67
Polar Electro company, 88, 94
President's Council on Physical Fit-
    ness and Sports, 42, 43
preventive medicine, 30–31
Prime Mover (Vogel), 120
Prior, Trevor, 253–54
pronation control, 254
Pruden, Bonnie, 42, 43
PTS (Personal Trainer System), 255
Puffer, James C., 72
purposive exercise, 37

Race Across America, 136–37
Radford, Peter, 33, 34, 35, 39
Rasch, Philip, 213
Reebok company, 48
Reeves, Steve, 212
Regimen in Health (Hippocrates),
    31
Reich, John, 4

Reiner, Carl, 222
Rendell, Hans, 114–15
*Research Quarterly for Exercise and
    Sport*, 66
Reynolds, Burt, 226
Ribisl, Paul, 159
Richardson, Benjamin Ward, 52–53,
    54–55
Richardson, Ron, 110–11
Ripping Gel, 256
Robertson, Brian, 106–7
Rome, Lawrence, 120–23, 232, 256–
    57
Roosevelt, Theodore, 39–40
rowing, 116
Rudder, Jeff, 149–50
runner's high, 172–73; addiction to
    exercise and, 175, 177–79, 186,
    192–97; endorphin hypothesis re-
    garding, 175–77, 188–91, 200;
    failure to achieve a high, 184–86;
    genetics of, 191–92, 196; heart rate
    and, 180; neurobiology of, 194–97;
    in rats, 192–94, 195–96; subjective
    experience of, 179–84; unknowns
    about, 186, 191
Runner's World magazine, 159
running, 29; aerobics and, 28; craze
    for, 46–48; heart-rate determina-
    tion with, 90; runner's high from,
    178–79; training for, 113–17; wa-
    gering contests, 33–35. *See also*
    marathon running

Salmons, Stanley, 124–26, 232
Saloff, David, 17–18
Sandow (Friedrich Mueller), 40
Schwartz, Kathryn, 102, 103, 135,
    139, 158, 168, 170, 181, 258
Schwarzenegger, Arnold, 225
Schwinn company, 253
scientific research, correct approach
    to, 261–62, 264–65
Seals, Douglas, 85–86, 87

self-improvement through exercise, 265–66
Self magazine, 4
serotonin, 186, 200
Sharkey, Brian J., 65
Sheehan, Andrew, 46
Sheehan, George, 26, 46–47, 224
shoes, 48, 253–54
Shorten, Martyn, 254
Silver, Lee, 182–83, 191, 192
Snyder, Solomon, 187–88, 189, 191
Solomon, Henry A., 60–61
Spa Lady gyms, 5–6, 205
Spinning, 6; cadence measure of effort, 78; certification of instructors, 243–45; conventions for instructors, 246–47; energy zones, 151; fan use during, 165; fat-burning zones and, 94–96; food intake for, 156, 158; heart rate and, 73, 77–79, 151; invention of, 135, 136–39; jumps, 141; marketing of, 253; master-presenter system, 150; mechanics of, 74–75; products associated with, 247; runner's high from, 93, 181–82; special-event rides, 7–8, 103–5, 140–41, 258–59; Taylor's experiences, 148–53; twelve-hour ride with Johnny G, 135–36, 139–40. *See also* Mount Everest ride
Spitzer, Marie, 39
Sports Club/LA company, 255
sports gels, 156, 158, 164
Sports Illustrated, 47, 222
Sports Medicine Advisory Committee, 19–20
stair-climbing machines, 48
Stampfl, Franz, 115
Starr, Bill, 220
Stefano, George, 12
Steinfeld, Jake, 226
steroids, 219–21, 223

Stockton, Pudgy and Les, 214–15
Strength & Health magazine, 210, 211, 212, 216, 220
stress tests, 57–58
stretching before exercise, 232
sugar and muscle fatigue, 162–64
SuperSlow exercise program, 250–52
sweating, 165
swimming, 262; aerobics and, 28; in cold water, 198; training for, 117, 118
Sydenham, Thomas, 186

Tanny, Vic, 211–12, 214
Taylor, Josh, 141–42, 143, 145–53, 155, 168, 169, 170, 171, 172, 258
Thom, Walter, 35–36
Thompson, Paul, 53–54, 71–72, 92, 227–28
Thompson, Tammy, 223
Tilney, Frederick, 216
Title IX, 226
Todd, Jan, 37, 38, 40, 41, 44, 208, 214–15, 217, 219, 221–23, 224, 225–26, 233
Todd, Terry, 221, 223
toning programs, 233–34
Tour de France, 54
training: base-building, 114; for bicycling, 107; cross-training, 105, 106; endurance training, 117–18; genetics of responsiveness to, 126–31; interval training, 105, 113–17, 129; for marathon running, 105–6, 107–13; for Mount Everest ride, 101–2, 155–58, 167; muscle physiology altered with, 119–26; over-training, diminishing returns from, 118–19; for pedestrianism, 35–36; purpose of, 118; for rowing, 116; for running, 113–17; for swimming, 117, 118; variety of approaches to, 105–13; for walking, 106–7
Travolta, John, 226

Vey, Randy, 166
VHA company, 16–17
Vogel, Steven, 120, 185, 209, 267

wagering contests, 32–35, 36, 39
Wainer, Howard, 15–16
walking, 29, 32, 62; health benefits, 262; training for, 106–7; wagering contests, 33–35, 36; weight control and, 3–4
warming up before exercise, 232
warm temperatures, exercising in, 166
water needs for exercise, 164–65, 166
wave communication, 18
Weider, Ben, 216
Weider, Joe, 215–17, 225
weight control, 69–70, 265; endorphins and, 175–76; fat-burning zones, 73, 80, 93–99; food intake and, 96–97; physics of, 96; walking and, 3–4; weight lifting and, 230–32
weight lifting, 200–201; attire for, 206; beginning a program, 263; behavior and communication among participants, 205–6; bodybuilding/bodysculpting, 203–5, 207, 208–9, 213–17, 219, 225; decline of sport weight lifting, 217–19; equipment for, 207; health benefits, 263, 265; health-club movement and, 226–27; Hoffman's career, 209–13; Hoffman-Weider conflict, 217, 219; homosexuals, association with, 219; metabolism and, 230–32; for Mount Everest ride, 155–56; Muscle Beach phenomenon, 213–15; as mythology for some people, 236–37; nutritional supplements, 210, 212–13, 256–57; osteoporosis and, 229–30; pain from, 205–6; pleasure of, 200, 207–9; poster boys for, 211–12; rules and pre-

scriptions for, 234–36; science of building muscles, 227–29; steroids and, 219–21, 223; strength training for athletes in other sports, 224–26; SuperSlow program, 250–52; toning programs, 233–34; types of lifts, 155–56, 218–19; Weider's career, 215–17; weight control and, 230–32; by women, 208–9, 211, 214–15, 221–24, 226, 227, 233–34
Weindruch, Larry, 48
West, Mae, 214
Weston, Edward P., 36
White, Paul Dudley, 60
Whorton, James C., 37, 52, 53
Wilkinson, Mary, 34
Williams, Harold, 55
Wilmore, Jack, 89, 98, 99, 227, 230–31
Wise, Roy, 188, 192, 194–95
Wohlford, Josephine, 38
women: heart effects of exercise, 63–64; in history of exercise and fitness, 34, 37–39, 40–41, 43–44, 45; weight lifting by, 208–9, 211, 214–15, 221–24, 226, 227, 233–34
World Gym, 214
Wyndham, C. H., 166–67

YogaButt exercise program, 247
York Barbell Company, 210
York Gang, 210, 211
Your Physique magazine, 215

Zapotek, Emil, 108, 109
Zenda, Phyllis, 247–48
Ziegler, John, 220
Zinkin, Harold, 214
Zoloft, 198–200
Zone Perfect company, 147
Zwick, Dan, 70

A NOTE ABOUT THE AUTHOR

Science reporter for *The New York Times*, Gina Kolata is the author of four previous books, most recently, *Flu: The Story of the Great Influenza Pandemic of 1918 and the Search for the Virus That Caused It* (FSG, 1999). She has been the recipient of numerous awards for her work, including an award from the American Medical Writers Association, the Susan G. Komen Foundation's media award for reporting on women's issues and breast cancer, and the 1995 award by the American Mathematics Association for reporting on mathematics; and, in 2000, she was a Pulitzer Prize finalist in investigative reporting. She lives in Princeton, New Jersey, where she and her husband spend much of their spare time exercising, as do their son and daughter.